JANELLA
PURCELL'S

elixir

JANELLA PURCELL'S

elixir

how to use food as medicine

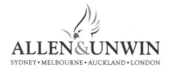

ALLEN&UNWIN
SYDNEY•MELBOURNE•AUCKLAND•LONDON

This book is intended as a source of information, not as a medical reference book. The reader is advised not to attempt self-treatment for serious or long-term problems without consulting a health professional.

Neither the author nor the publisher can be held responsible for any adverse reactions to the recipes, recommendations and instructions contained in the book and the use of any ingredient is entirely at the reader's own risk.

First published in 2004

Allen & Unwin
Sydney, Melbourne, Auckland, London

83 Alexander Street
Crows Nest NSW 2065
Australia
Phone: (61 2) 8425 0100
Email: info@allenandunwin.com
Web: www.allenandunwin.com

Cataloguing-in-Publication details are available
from the National Library of Australia
www.trove.nla.gov.au

ISBN 978 1 74331 490 6

Set in 11/16 pt Sabon LT Pro by Bookhouse, Sydney
Printed in Australia by Ligare Book Printers, Australia

10 9 8 7 6 5 4 3 2 1

elixir /əˈlɪksə / *n.* **1.** sovereign remedy; panacea; cure for all. **2.** the quintessence or absolute embodiment of anything. **3.** preparation believed to prolong life. **4.** fragrant liquid used as a medicine or flavouring. **5.** a remedy believed to cure all ills.

Contents

Introduction

It's been almost a decade since I wrote *Elixir*. In this time I have learnt so much more about using food as medicine that I thought it was time for a second edition. So here it is, complete with new entries such as coconut, cacao, goji berries, cellulite and sustainably caught seafood. I've loved updating *Elixir*. I hope you enjoy the new information. Who knows, maybe the third edition in another decade . . .

For me, there is no doubt that the food you eat affects your health and your state of mind. Even the most natural foods could make you sick simply because you are not eating them correctly. Many people might disagree with me, but after a lifetime of study and practice there are few things of which I am more sure.

Early in life everyone develops eating patterns that become habitual. The connection between love, emotional bonding and food are common to most cultures. These habits become deeply ingrained and may lead to disease later in our lives. Most people are unaware of their true appetite due to regularly over-eating—they don't let their bodies experience hunger. Their bodies have forgotten how to digest properly due to a lack of appetite and chewing, and/or eating too quickly. For example, when someone is stressed, either emotionally or physically, their stomach shuts down, making digestion and absorption of nutrients almost impossible. This is a time when you shouldn't eat difficult to digest food, such as animal products and grains. Simple broths or miso are recommended and juices are also effective.

Your dietary needs change not only from season to season but also with the seasons of your life. When you are younger, you need a diet higher in nutrients such as protein and oil to support growth. As an adult your dietary requirements change due to your metabolism (and usually your activity levels) slowing down. You now need a diet high in fibre—a diet for maintenance.

Another issue that has arisen in today's busy society is that home cooking has been put on the 'back burner', because it is considered too time-consuming. This is unhealthy because the alternative to home cooking is usually fast food. Fast foods are often prepared with products that contribute to disease—transfatty acids, substandard produce and more fat than is suggested in the daily allowance recommended by nutritionists. Hence the greater number of obese people and the higher incidence of diabetes in our society. This is more than a shame and it is avoidable because once you know the basic principles of healthy cooking, the possibilities are endless and easy. If you explore and enjoy the food you eat, ultimately it will become you. You are what you eat.

The energetics of food

A Western understanding of food is dependent upon the laboratory, upon the analysis and breakdown of food into its basic components. In the West, food is described as possessing certain quantities of nutrients—protein, iron, vitamins etc. Eastern understanding is derived from the observation of human behaviour once food is taken into the body. Not unlike modern physics, the world is seen in terms of energy and vibration. Some foods activate your metabolism, some foods slow you down; some foods generate warmth in the body, some coolness; some foods are moistening, some drying; some nourish your kidneys, others your heart or liver.

One of the basic principles of eating under this philosophy is to eat according to who *you* are. There is no such thing as a universally applicable 'right' diet. A person is described as a combination of certain basic qualities such as hot, cold, dry or moist. Each food has qualities that make it what it is. Among the qualities of food, the temperature is the most important. This doesn't mean you eat it when it's hot or cold temperature-wise, instead it is a measure of the effect the food has on your metabolism after initial digestion—its energetic temperature. Cucumbers, tomatoes and yoghurt, for example, are at the cooling end, while capsicums, lamb and garlic are up at the warming end. Other foods—such as sardines, cabbage, organic tofu and grapes—are considered neutral. Many traditional recipes reflect an underlying understanding of the energetic principles of balancing food—for example, the combinations lamb and mint sauce, beef and horseradish, and lettuce and cheese.

A primarily hot person will need to eat a mostly cooling diet, plenty of fruit and vegetables, fish instead of meat, and not too many spicy or fatty foods. Alcohol and coffee are heating substances so they should be avoided if you are already hot, or during summer. A cool person will need a more warming diet—plenty of stews and casseroles and warming ingredients such as ginger and garlic. They also need to avoid cooling substances such as tea or raw foods.

When you are ill, a simple cure may be in your kitchen. A hot, acute illness when you are restless, feverish, inflamed and perhaps have a sore throat or high temperature may be helped by a cup of peppermint tea or by a simple, thin vegetable soup of zucchini, celery or carrot. Conversely, it may be made worse by hot foods such as Thai or Mexican cuisines, or congesting foods such as meat and dairy. If your illness is more cold in nature with shivering, aches and a desire to curl up with a hot water, the opposite principle can be applied—ginger tea or a thin onion soup. Cold foods such as fruit or salad will slow down the recovery in this instance.

The flavour of food tells us more about its action. There are five basic flavours—sweet, pungent, salty, sour and bitter—and each of these will benefit a particular organ and carry out certain actions.

The energetics of food reveals the potential effects food might have on the body, mind and spirit of the person consuming it. The following are examples of how foods are classified.

Asparagus
Flavour Sweet and bitter
Function Cooling
Indications Constipation, hypertension, high cholesterol, diabetes, bronchitis

Lemon
Flavour Sour
Function Cold
Indications Cough

Ginger
Flavour Pungent
Function Warm
Indications Dysentery

Tofu
Flavour Bland
Function Neutral
Indications Dry cough

Coffee
Flavour Bitter
Function Hot
Indications Stimulates the liver

The way you cook your food will affect its vitality, and different methods are suited to different individuals. It is important to know when associating a food with a particular energy that it can be altered through food preparation methods. For example, roasting is warming; salads are cleansing and cooling; steaming and boiling are neutral; and stir-frying is a little more warming than steaming. Adding ginger or garlic or other warming spices makes the food warmer and therefore easier to digest.

Organic, biodynamic or genetically modified-free foods have stronger and more health-giving energetic structures than commercially grown, over-watered and chemically fed food. The energetic structure of food is also severely weakened by the use of microwaves. The importance of quality food cannot be stressed enough, and fortunately more and more people are realising this. We need to keep balance in mind. This is achieved by eating in moderation and by being aware of tastes and variety. If we eat a balanced diet with many tastes, then we feel satisfied and won't want to binge immediately after a meal.

about this book

In addition to understanding the energetics of food, there are three elements that underpin my philosophy towards food and its health-giving properties. The first is the benefits to be found in the foods in the Japanese diet. Bancha tea, umeboshi plums, kombu, the other sea vegetables, miso—these foods have greatly contributed to the longevity of the Japanese people. I strongly urge you to incorporate them into your diet; you will find ways to do so throughout this book.

Second, as you may have guessed, I believe the *way* you eat is vitally important. For example, chewing your food well will make it less acidic, therefore easier to digest, absorb and assimilate/use. The third strong belief I have is the use of food as an alternative to conventional medicine and as a preventative to disease. Modern medicine has so many side effects that the use of nature's abundant store of health-enhancing goodies is just commonsense.

This book is an A to Z, so you'll easily find the topics that will be of interest to you specifically. If you are diabetic you'll look at the *Diabetes, type 2* entry. Of course, if you are not, you may not read it but I suggest you do as the information is as much about preventing the onset of the disease as controlling it through food. To gain the most benefit, read the whole book and keep it handy for future reference.

At the back you will find a list of herbs and the table outlining the energetics of food. I hope you enjoy this book as much as I have enjoyed putting it together for you. Remember, prevention is better than cure, so invest some time and thought in your health to reap the most from your life. Live well.

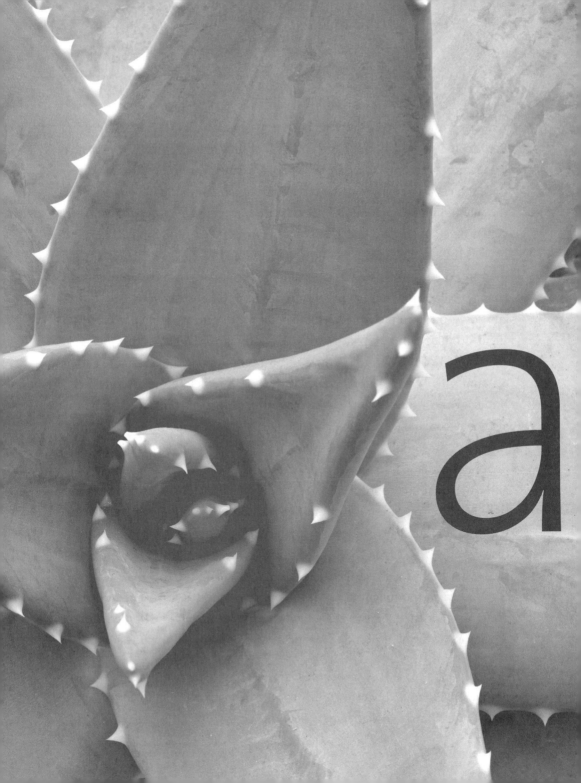

a

ACIDOSIS

Acidosis is an imbalance between body acids and alkalis—there is an increase in the activity of the body's fluid and tissues. Too much acidity is responsible for many health complaints, including gout, ageing, frozen shoulder and digestive problems. To counteract it, you should eat mostly alkaline foods—that is, they should make up about 80 per cent of your diet. The problem, however, is that much of the Western diet comes from acid-forming foods. The good news is that, by chewing your food well, adding kombu to your beans while they are cooking and using umeboshi plum products, you have a pretty good chance of keeping your acidity to a minimum. Of course, you also need to cut down on extremely acidic foods—dairy, red meat, refined wheat and sugar products, and all processed foods—if not avoid them altogether.

The pH of the human body is naturally mildly acidic, sitting between 6.0 and 6.8. Water is considered neutral at 7.0. Below 6.3 is considered acidic, while values above 6.8 are alkaline. (Special pH paper, which is available from a chemist, will allow you to test your level of pH and change your diet accordingly.) Diabetics tend to suffer from acidosis, caused by such factors as kidney, liver or adrenal disorders; obesity; stress, such as anger and fear; and an inappropriate diet. Symptoms of acidosis include frequent sighing, water retention, insomnia, migraines, low blood pressure, trouble with swallowing, sensitive teeth and alternating constipation and diarrhoea. Listed below are foods that are strongly acid- and alkaline-forming and those that are almost neutral.

Naturally, too much stress will only add to the amount of acid in your body, so mindful exercises that involve deep breathing and some form of meditation will be extremely beneficial in balancing your body.

Acid-forming foods

Alcohol, asparagus, beans, brussels sprouts, chickpeas, cocoa, coffee, eggs, fish, white flour and its products, legumes, meat (including organs), milk, mustard, oats, olives, pepper, plums, poultry, prunes, shellfish, soft drinks, sugar and its products, tea and vinegar. Also acid-forming are most drugs (prescription and recreational) and tobacco.

Alkaline-forming foods

Avocados, corn, dates, fresh coconut, most fruits and vegetables (citrus are alkaline-forming), honey, maple syrup, molasses, raisins, sea vegetables and soybeans and their products.

Almost neutral foods

Buckwheat, butter, canned fruit, cheese, chestnuts, dried fruit (mostly), grains (mostly), ice cream, lima beans, millet, seeds and nuts (mostly).

See also SEA VEGETABLES and UMEBOSHI PRODUCTS.

AGAR AGAR

Refer to SEA VEGETABLES.

AMARANTH

This is one of the oldest cereal varieties cultivated by humans and the principal foodstuff of the Incas and Aztecs. It is extraordinarily healthy as a cereal or foliage plant because of its high protein content—16 per cent. It also contains loads of fibre, amino acids and vitamin C, and it has more calcium, magnesium and silicon than milk. It is higher in lysine, an essential amino acid, than other grains.

Amaranth is great for those with increased nutritional needs such as lactating mums, pregnant women, children, toddlers and those who do physical work. It has an intense flavour (and is quite pricey), so it may be mixed with other grains. Available as a grain, puffs, flour and flakes, it is gluten-free.

See also WHOLEGRAINS.

AMASAKE

Amasake is fermented sweet rice. A starter called koji, which has been treated with a yeast culture called *Aspergillus oryzae*, has converted the starch in rice into a simple sugar. This sugar is not refined, as it is not as concentrated as honey, molasses etc.

ANTI-AGEING

Many of us are afraid to grow old and one reason may be the way our Western society deals with and views the elderly. Other cultures value and respect their elders, and rightly so. The wisdom accumulated from living to a ripe old age is there for the more youthful to learn from—as the old saying goes, 'Youth is wasted on the young'.

Another reason we fear old age might be the supposed lack of independence due to declining health or stamina. There is no need for you to view old age and disease as inseparable. Staying vital through old age has a lot to do with good dietary practices and attitude. Digestive abilities do decrease as you age, so the food you eat as well as your eating habits are important at this time in your life. Equally important are those practices that deepen spiritual awareness. Techniques such as tai qi, yoga and meditation are extremely beneficial throughout your life, especially in the 'winter' years.

You need to keep your mind and body active throughout your life, and the earlier you start, the healthier you will be as you age.

Helpful foods for longevity and during old age

🌿 leafy green vegetables, especially locally sourced sea vegetables (kelp, dunaliella, nori, arame and wakame), barley and wheatgrass products, which are gluten-free and packed with more minerals than any other food, help reverse the effects of refined sugar, which devastates the mineral condition of the body

- complex carbohydrates—wholegrains, fruits and vegetables, legumes, nuts and seeds—are fibre-rich foods that clean the heart and arteries and keep the digestive tract functioning smoothly
- sprouts of any kind are good for breaking down fats, protein and starches, making them easier to digest
- millet, barley (try it in soup), organic tofu, black soybeans, mung beans, locally sourced sea vegetables and spirulina moisten the body, so they can help if you tend to suffer from constipation
- black sesame seeds and flaxseed oil are also great for moistening the intestines, making bowel movements smoother
- almonds, avocado and coconut—great sources of essential fatty acids—are good for those who tend to be thin, dry, anxious and nervous
- organic chicken broth or mussels (a good form of sustainably caught seafood)—according to traditional Chinese medicine, these help with senility or depression.

Foods to avoid

- acidic foods—refined sugar products, coffee, alcohol, too much refined salt and highly processed foods, including white flour, biscuits, pasta, bread and sugar—as they weaken the entire body and prevent proper calcium absorption. Instead of refined white sugar try rice syrup, agave, coconut palm sugar, rapadura (panela), molasses, spelt syrup, maple syrup or raw honey
- excessive amounts of salt, as it will increase blood pressure and inhibit mineral uptake from other foods
- too much animal protein, as this will cause calcium loss and put increased pressure on your body, especially the organs that aid digestion, respiration and circulation—if you want or feel as if you need a

bit of meat in your later years, make it organic organ meat, marrow, fish or meat broth, as these are easier on your digestive organs

- dairy products, because lactose intolerance increases with age and they are high in fat; fermented dairy products (yoghurt, quark and some cottage cheese) are usually best. For the heavier older person and those with a high-fat dietary background, reduce or avoid dairy altogether, although (organic) goat products are lower in fat and easier to digest.

Herbal medicine

- *Ginkgo biloba* has been shown in clinical studies to increase blood flow and neural transmission to the brain. Ginkgo, the oldest living tree species, may reduce symptoms such as memory loss, vertigo, ringing in the ears and depression
- rehmannia, used for adrenal exhaustion, aids in the functioning of your kidneys
- withania is a lovely herb for your adrenal glands, thereby increasing energy and decreasing anxiety; it's also useful after you've been sick and/or depleted
- licorice is another good adrenal herb, plus it helps to curb sugar cravings as well as aids easier bowel movements.

Supplements

- royal jelly and bee pollen (check for allergy) contain almost all the nutrients your body requires, as they are complete foods packed with essential nutrients. They are used for convalescence, to increase vitality and endurance. They also improve immunity. Use these products mindfully as they are the bees' food
- kelp, spirulina, wheat and barley grasses are packed with important enzymes and help your liver to eliminate fat and toxins
- magnesium and calcium, together, for cardiovascular health, bone density and nervous system, and also to aid sleep.

Lifestyle factors

- avoid over-eating, as this is the major cause of ageing in wealthier countries—eat until you are two-thirds full only
- do not eat late at night—eat the last meal of the day as early as possible and make it small, easy to digest and nourishing
- avoid fad diets and products and make any dietary changes gradually, facilitated by a healthcare practitioner
- eat foods that are easy to digest—miso, purées and blended soups may be necessary for those who have difficulty chewing.

See also ARTHRITIS, MEMORY, PROSTATE and ZINC.

APHRODISIACS

Food and sex have been linked for centuries and are still intimately entwined. They both ensure the survival of the human race, and both provide opportunities for fun. Maybe this is why foods that stimulate the libido have been part of our lives for thousands of years. Or is it because giving and receiving pleasure may be life-extending?

Almost any food can ignite passion if it's prepared and eaten with love in mind. Given the opportunity, practically no one would reject a sensual, warm feeling throughout their body. Food can remind us of sex because of its taste, texture or appearance. In this way food is an aphrodisiac, arousing our desires.

Aphrodisiacs work on many levels, based on chemical, sensory, emotional, romantic and social factors. When you eat or cook, you use the same senses you do when making love—smell, touch, taste, sight and hearing. Sex is a balance between expansive (male or yang) forces and contractive (yin or female) forces. Aphrodisiacs work in the same way—for example, champagne (yin) and caviar (yang).

It is important to be aware of your mood when you are preparing a meal, as those emotions will be imparted into the dish, like it or not. Every meal is an opportunity to come together and toast sex, love, romance, family and life. Sadly this has become less important in our lives, maybe because we weren't taught how to prepare and serve a meal or because there doesn't seem to be enough time. Whatever the case, below are some foods that will turn you and your lover on without too much preparation time. 'Make love not war.'

Asparagus In nineteenth-century France, bridegrooms were required to eat several courses consisting of asparagus because of its reputed powers to arouse.

Basil This herb is still used in voodoo love ceremonies in Haiti.

Cardamom According to traditional Indian herbal medicine, a nightcap of powdered cardamom boiled with milk and mixed with honey can cure impotence and premature ejaculation.

Dates In Iran dates are used to help people whose sex life is less than satisfying.

Eggs For centuries eggs have been regarded as fertility symbols, perhaps because they represent new life.

Figs The fig has the reputation of being one of the sexiest fruits on the planet, probably due to its many seeds and 'pear shape'. A variety of the *Ficus* tree, which is thought to have originated in Asia, is one of the oldest known edible plants.

Grapes In Greek mythology, Dionysus was the god of wine as well as fertility and procreation. Grapes, which have been eaten by humans since Neolithic times, are his symbol.

Honey Sweet and spreadable, honey makes an ideal love food. The word 'honeymoon' derives from an ancient custom requiring newlyweds to lick mead (honey wine) off each other's palms for the first lunar month after marriage to ensure a sweet life together. The Egyptians also regarded honey as a lover's treat and offered it to the god of fertility.

Ice cream Another favourite love food, ice cream arouses because of its 'smearing' potential.

Java This is a coffee and, like all coffees (in moderation), it stimulates the senses.

Kumquats This is an unusual and sensual fruit. Put a whole kumquat in your mouth, then bite—the citrus explosion will excite your taste buds.

Licorice This delicacy increases blood pressure, thereby sending blood to the penis, aiding erection.

Mango An exotic and sensual fruit, mango has a moist flesh; a massage with its skin is very erotic.

Nutmeg This fragrant spice has long been prized as an aphrodisiac by Arabs, Greeks, Hindus and Romans. In India a combination of nutmeg, honey and a half-boiled egg is eaten an hour before sex to prolong lovemaking.

Onions For thousands of years onions have been used as an aphrodisiac. They are recommended in both ancient Hindu and Arabic texts on the art of making love. In France, newlyweds are served onion soup the day after their wedding to restore sexual vigour, and priests in ancient Egypt (and others who took their spiritual practice very seriously) abstained from onions because they were reputed to increase libido.

Oysters Legend has it that Casanova ate 50 raw oysters every morning in the bathtub—he used a beautiful woman's breast as his plate. Oysters are high in zinc, and medical research has found that a low sperm count and libido can be connected to low zinc levels.

Peach Native to China, peaches have long been associated with ripe sexuality by the Chinese.

Pomegranate This deep red-coloured fruit is recommended in the *Karma Sutra* as an erotic aid.

Quinces Due to its colour and many seeds, the quince was dedicated to Aphrodite, the Greek goddess of love. Quince is eaten at some weddings to ensure a sweet life for the newly married couple. Some also say the quince, not the apple, was the fruit that tempted Eve.

Rice This symbol of fertility is a staple food in Asia. In some cultures if a man and woman eat out of the same rice bowl it is a declaration of their engagement. Rice is thrown at wedding ceremonies for good luck and the possibility of many children.

Saffron This spice has been reputed to work like a sex hormone and make erogenous zones even more sensitive. Saffron is made from the dried stigmas of a type of crocus. Each crocus has about three stigmas, which must be picked by hand. About 225 000 stigmas are needed to make half a kilogram of saffron, which is why this spice is highly prized.

Tomatoes There's nothing more sensuous than watching a true Italian lovingly preparing tomatoes, known as love apples by the French, for a rich sauce.

Unagi (raw eel) This popular Japanese aphrodisiac is used in sushi, which is a great love food, thanks to the erotic Japanese film, *In the Realm of the Senses* (1976).

Vanilla The word 'vanilla' comes from the Spanish word *vaina*, which means 'vagina'. It is a powerful aphrodisiac. Try dabbing a little vanilla on your wrists, or draw a bath for two scented with real vanilla extract.

Walnuts In Rome, walnuts were thrown at newlyweds instead of rice and also used in ancient fertility ceremonies. Walnuts have also been used in Italy and France to intensify desire.

Xanat This flower from the vanilla plant was named after the youngest daughter of a South American fertility goddess. According to legend, the daughter transformed herself into a plant that would bring pleasure and happiness.

Yohimbe This herb increases blood flow to the penis by increasing testosterone, hence libido.

Zinc Linked to fertility, sexual desire and potency, men and women who have low zinc levels may also have a decreased sex drive.

ARAME

This sea vegetable contains ten times more calcium than milk does and 500 times more iodine than shellfish.

See also SEA VEGETABLES.

ARTHRITIS

The surfaces of the bones that meet at the joints are covered with a layer of cartilage and surrounded by a capsule made up of ligaments. Inside this capsule is fluid, which is responsible for allowing the bones to glide past one another without friction. When the smooth surface of cartilage covering the ends of the bones becomes rough over time, it causes friction. This degenerative joint disease is called osteoarthritis. It is sometimes caused by an injury, but more often it is due to the wear and tear of ageing.

Symptoms of osteoarthritis can be pain, swelling, stiffness and/or decreased movement. The swelling can be the result of an increase in fluid, thickening of the membranes, enlargement of the bones or a combination of these. Arthritis typically runs in families and affects three times more women than men.

Helpful foods

- alkaline foods, such as umeboshi plums, vegetables, sprouts, cereal grasses, locally sourced sea vegetables and herbs; too much acid in your blood will cause the cartilage to dissolve, causing the joints to lose their smooth, gliding action so the bones rub together and the joints become inflamed

- omega 3 foods, such as mackerel, anchovies and sardines—try to eat deep-sea, cold-water fish three to five times a week. (Eat sustainably caught fish only and avoid tuna due to its heavy metal levels and decreasing numbers.)
- once converted in the gut, flaxseed oil contains very high levels of omega 3, as do chia seeds and walnuts; all three have strong anti-inflammatory properties
- avocado, olive oil, green tea, goats milk, chlorophyll, macadamias, ginger and turmeric are good anti-inflammatory foods
- alfalfa is a time-honoured remedy for bone disorders such as arthritis
- use spelt and kamut (ancient grains) instead of refined wheat—buy spelt pasta and kamut bread, for example
- eat quinoa instead of white rice and couscous
- soy, broccoli, radish or snow pea sprouts, for their high content of nutrients, including chlorophyll
- cooked cabbage for digestion, beetroot for building blood, celery for fluid retention and shallots to 'cool' the system
- chives—drink as a tea or apply its leaves to the arthritic area
- foods high in calcium, magnesium, chlorophyll and minerals—grains, legumes, leafy greens, cereal grasses and locally sourced sea vegetables (kelp, nori and wakame)
- umeboshi products (see *Umeboshi products*), as they are strong alka-lisers and wonderful for your digestion.

Foods to avoid

- animal fats, including dairy and red and white meat (organic chicken may be eaten one to three times a week)
- processed and refined wheat and its products
- processed and refined oils, including margarine and trans fats
- junk food

- coffee (especially instant) and too much alcohol and refined sugar
- too many warming foods such as garlic and hot spices
- the Nightshade family of vegetables—including capsicum, white potatoes, tomatoes, eggplant and chillies (these are neutralised somewhat by cooking with salt or miso, and red potatoes have the mildest effect)—inhibits calcium absorption, is acid-forming and increases arthritis pain
- citrus fruits
- calcium inhibitors—alcohol, coffee, marijuana, excess meat and other protein, refined sugar and excess salt. Rhubarb, cranberries, plums and silver beet are fine in moderation, so eat them when they are in season.

Herbal medicine

- boswellia for inflammation involved with arthritic pain
- devil's claw for pain when treating arthritis
- celery for fluid retention around joints
- ginger for relief from muscular aches and pain and to increase circulation
- cat's claw and echinacea, both immune modulators
- turmeric, a great anti-inflammatory
- St John's wort for pain and general inflammation
- willow bark (the source of aspirin) for any pain
- dandelion root for good liver health
- gotu kola (pennywort), an anti-inflammatory, is known to relieve the pain of rheumatism and arthritis.

Supplements

- glucosamine and chondroitin for cartilage repair and growth (you can buy these together as a powder); many orthopaedic surgeons are prescribing these now instead of corticosteroids
- calcium and magnesium, taken together for healthy bones
- zinc, a good antioxidant, for bone growth and immune response
- flaxseed oil, an anti-inflammatory that helps with pain

- vitamin C for its anti-inflammatory effect; it also helps with pain, bruising and circulation
- spirulina, wheat and barley grasses and kelp, as they will help the liver process toxins and fats; they are also packed with enzymes
- royal jelly (check for allergy)—a great immune booster that contains essential nutrients; use it mindfully.

Lifestyle factors

- get regular and moderate exercise—walking, swimming, bike riding and watersports are good choices; avoid weight-bearing or impact exercises
- reduce your weight—those extra kilos can cause and aggravate symptoms
- avoid non-steroidal anti-inflammatory drugs (NSAIDs) as the side effects—such as stomach ulcers, gastrointestinal (gut) bleeding and kidney or liver damage—are very common
- Drink alkaline water. Don't drink tap water, especially if it's been fluoridated, as it can lead to brittle bones and kidney problems.

Essential oils

- ginger can be used in a massage oil to improve blood circulation and decrease pain—mix together ten drops of ginger oil, three drops of rosemary and juniper oils and ½ cup sesame oil
- sesame oil specifically is good for relieving the pain of arthritis.

See also ACIDOSIS, ANTI-AGEING, CALCIUM and PULSES (LEGUMES).

ASIAN CUISINE

Low in saturated fat and high in protein, calcium and iron, Asian cuisine is a desirable diet. Knowing how to use the ingredients for this diet, however, seems to be where people experience problems. Asian supermarkets and the Asian sections in health food stores and supermarkets often intimidate shoppers with their unfamiliar products. But inside these stores you will

Miso soup

I like to eat miso soup when I'm feeling a bit flat, tired and hungry but don't feel like eating because I'm feeling anxious, or under the weather for whatever reason. This is probably the dish I eat most.

SERVES 4

4–6 shiitake mushrooms (as an immune booster and good source of vitamin B12)

½ bunch of coriander (as a digestive aid)

2–3 sachets of dashi (an Asian stock made from shiitake mushrooms, kombu and fish flakes)

½ daikon (white radish), diced (helps liver to process fats)

selection of vegetables, as desired

½ cup organic miso paste (protein)

2 tablespoons spring onions, finely sliced (balances energetics of meal)

½ sheet of nori, optional (for protein and calcium)

1   Fill a medium-sized soup pot with 4 litres of filtered water. Add the shiitake mushrooms and finely chopped coriander root, reserving leaves for garnish. Bring to the boil. When soft, remove mushrooms from the pot. Remove stems of mushrooms and discard (or save for making a stock). Slice mushrooms finely and put back in the pot along with the dashi.

2   Add daikon and any other vegetables you'd like—the more vegetables, the thicker the soup. Cook until the vegetables are soft. When ready, turn off the heat and stir in the miso but don't let it boil.

3   Serve in individual bowls topped with finely sliced spring onions, reserved coriander leaves and shredded nori, if using.

find highly valued food secrets that have held the key to healthy living for thousands of years. These ingredients are simple to use, cheap and highly nutritious. Remember, however, that most soy products are genetically modified, so you must choose organic products. In addition, you will usually find many additives in packaged Asian foods. Look at the label to check they haven't added numbers, especially those staring with 'e'. Monosodium glutamate (MSG), for example, is e621. You also don't want sugar of any kind. Finally, check out the product's origin—don't buy products from Japan due to the devastating and toxic nuclear fallout from the earthquake at Fukushima.

See also BANCHA TEA, OESTROGEN, SEA VEGETABLES, SOY PRODUCTS and UMEBOSHI PRODUCTS.

ASTHMA

Asthma can be difficult to diagnose, as it resembles a number of other diseases, such as bronchitis, emphysema and lower respiratory infections. This disease causes obstruction of the airways, which are usually hypersensitive to certain allergens or stimuli.

Common allergens	Other triggers
Cats and feathers	Adrenal exhaustion
Chemicals	Dryness or humidity
Drugs	Low blood sugar
Dust mites	Exercise
Environmental pollutants	Stress
Food additives	Fear and anxiety
Mould	Change of temperature
Tobacco smoke	Laughing

We tend not to breathe correctly when we are upset—we usually take short breaths—which may be why traditional Chinese medicine says that problems with the lungs are associated with the emotions of grief and sadness.

Helpful foods

- apricots (sulfur-free) to calm panting and ease attack—also good for a dry cough as they moisten the lungs
- kelp to soothe the lungs and ease attack
- daikon (white radish) to ease a raspy cough
- persimmons moisten the lungs, so they are good for the coughing and wheezing associated with asthma; **avoid** in cases of diarrhoea
- walnuts are warming and calming for asthmatic lungs
- black soybeans relieve coughing
- fresh ginger will reduce inflammation in the lungs
- fresh fruit and vegetables should make up the bulk of an asthmatic's diet as these foods are high in essential vitamins, minerals and fibre
- a diet relatively high in plant protein and low in refined carbohydrates, as they quickly turn to sugar—protein is needed for rebuilding damaged cells
- garlic and onions are anti-inflammatory (use in moderation only)
- raw goats milk is usually okay as it is anti-inflammatory and alkaline-forming
- foods rich in vitamin A and chlorophyll to process toxins through the liver—such as kale, carrots, pumpkin, spirulina, apricots, goji berries and leafy green vegetables—as they are antioxidants and immune-boosting
- pumpkin promotes discharge of mucus from the lungs
- raw turnip and radish (try grating and sprinkling with umeboshi vinegar) to disperse lung congestion and mucus
- kale eases lung congestion
- almonds alleviate coughs and disperse phlegm
- omega 3 oils from fish such as blue eye cod and mackerel as well as pumpkin, flaxseed and chia seeds, leafy green vegetables and walnuts

- warming foods, such as pine nuts, anchovies, mussels, walnuts, chestnuts, turtle and adzuki beans, and lentils for depletion—these foods will keep your blood running smoothly around your body. Adding rosemary to these legumes will make them even warmer and tastier.

Foods to avoid

- refined sugar and artificial sweeteners will demineralise your system
- cold foods, as they will shock your bronchioles
- animal fats such as lamb, and beef and dairy foods are inflammatory and acidic, making allergic conditions worse
- peanuts, as many people are allergic to them
- too much of warming spices such as cinnamon and fennel may constrict bronchioles
- dairy
- refined wheat is often a problem, as it is an inflammatory food that goes rancid soon after it is ground.

Herbal medicine

- *Ginkgo biloba* for persistent asthma
- boswellia, an anti-inflammatory for the respiratory tract
- baical skullcap, an anti-allergic
- albizia, an anti-allergic
- licorice, an anti-inflammatory for the lungs—in cases of high blood pressure, avoid it
- cat's claw for immune-boosting
- mullein, a respiratory tonic
- ginger for circulation and inflammation
- horsetail for long-term lung weakness

- golden seal for inflammation in the mucous membranes
- St Mary's thistle, dandelion root or schisandra for the liver.

Supplements

- lotus root powder will help any respiratory problem; mix it with honey to make a tea
- vitamin B12 will decrease lung inflammation
- kelp relieves coughing and asthma
- magnesium and calcium as muscle relaxants; magnesium to aid calcium utilisation, and calcium to balance the magnesium
- vitamin C for inflammation
- flaxseed oil to decrease inflammation
- wheatgrass, spirulina or barley grass, packed with vitamin A, are antioxidants and immune boosters; they are also very high in protein and enzymes.

Lifestyle factors

- avoid air pollutants and dust mites
- avoid sulfite agents, which are often found in restaurant food such as shellfish, cut fruit and green salads
- eat light meals
- improve your digestion by chewing well
- avoid synthetic additives of any kind
- decrease stress and deal with any unresolved grief or sadness
- swim for exercise—it is better than running or walking, which both heat the body too much
- avoid tobacco
- all cleaning and body products—including air fresheners, makeup and hand soap—must be 100 per cent natural and organic.

Essential oils

- marjoram
- eucalyptus.

See also AUTUMN, COLDS AND 'FLU, ENERGY, HAYFEVER and
ORGANS AND ASSOCIATED EMOTIONS.

ATHLETES

One of the biggest problems facing athletes today is that they end up eating terrible food due to the heavy burden regular training places on the body. As their body uses up everything and still needs more, athletes invariably turn to protein powders and enormous amounts of synthetic supplementation. This is unhealthy, unnecessary, expensive and, in many cases, potentially dangerous. The right diet and rest are just as important as the right exercise regimen, and an appropriate balance of them all is ideal.

I don't support high-protein diets or protein powders. Athletes do have increased protein needs, but too much animal protein and synthetic powders can stress the kidneys and contribute to toxic waste in the colon and throughout the body. Below is a guide to where your nutrients should come from and in what quantities.

Carbohydrates (50–60% of total kilojoules)	Proteins (15–20%, max. 25%)	Fats (25–30%)
10–20% simple—fruits, most vegetables, any treats	Animal—fish, poultry, meats, eggs, dairy products (organic and sustainable)	Saturated (less than half)—meats, eggs, dairy products (organic and sustainable)
40–50% complex—whole-grains, legumes, starchy vegetables	Vegetable—nuts, seeds, legumes, sea vegetables, wheatgrass	Unsaturated (more than half)—nuts, seeds, vegetable oils, avocado

Helpful foods

- complex carbohydrates, including wholegrains and their products, such as wheat-free (or kamut or spelt) pasta, legumes, potatoes and other starchy vegetables; the body uses complex carbohydrates much more efficiently than other foods for its energy needs and stores them for later use
- quality vegetable protein instead of animal protein
- fruits (not always bananas) are very high in protein
- low to moderate amounts of unrefined oil or fat
- high-protein, low-fat foods such as fish and poultry are better than red meats
- nuts and seeds that are high in essential oils and protein, such as chia seed, flaxseed, almonds, brazil nuts and pistachios
- locally sourced sea vegetables are a fabulous source of low-fat protein
- miso paste, tempeh and locally sourced sea vegetables such as wakame, nori and arame are good vegetarian sources of easy-to-digest proteins—miso and sea vegetable soup is a prime example of a protein-, vitamin-, enzyme- and mineral-rich meal. It is easy to digest, as it has been pre-digested by bacterial action during fermentation[1]
- spirulina, chlorella and wild blue–green algae are the richest whole-food sources of protein—micro-algae are excellent building foods, as well as being good cleansers due to their chlorophyll content
- kamut, oats, spelt, quinoa and amaranth are high-protein grains that may be most suitable for those with a high-fat dietary background—the amount of protein in quinoa and amaranth is about the same as meat

---

1   Fermented foods supply protein and other nutrients in an easily digestible form as a result of predigestion by bacteria. Once the fermentation is complete, the micro-organisms remain in the food as mostly protein, but under the right conditions as vitamin B12.

and, when combined with another grain, their amino acid/protein profile is higher than meat or any other animal product.

Foods to avoid

- fatty foods such as fried foods, lunchmeats, bacon, ham and any foods cooked in animal fats—a high-fat diet is definitely out for athletes, as it slows them down and can increase body–fat percentage
- dairy
- excess protein, as it can produce clogging of the colon and put stress on the kidneys—protein is needed for tissue building and any excess must be used for energy or it will be eliminated.

Herbal medicine

- ginseng root has been known to increase stamina
- cayenne pepper is a natural stimulant that may raise the metabolism and increase energy levels
- silicon or silica, usually derived from the herb horsetail, is important for elasticity and flexibility in the tissues
- damiana has a testosterone-like action, so it will increase energy (and libido)
- Siberian ginseng, sage, rosehip, lemonbalm and damiana as a tea will benefit any physical or mental performance—brew and drink on the morning of the event.

Supplements

- amino acid formulas can be used to increase protein levels, as can pea-based protein powders
- iron is especially important for female athletes
- spirulina and chlorella, as they are two of the best sources of protein.

Lifestyle factors

- drink water a couple of hours before an event to hydrate the body's tissues, and during an event if there is extended competition—dehydration from low fluid intake leads to weakened tissue perfusion (circulation of blood with oxygen and nutrients), fatigue and poor performance. Include enough alkaline water and coconut water
- for fluid replacement it is best to avoid salty and sugary drinks, lots of fruit juices and artificially sweetened drinks. For long events, add a little sweet liquid such as fruit juice to the water to provide some kilojoules and energy. Or try adding chlorophyll and coconut water
- avoid alcohol, smoking and stimulants, such as caffeine in coffee, tea and cola beverages
- when training is reduced, the food you eat needs to be altered—you need to consume fewer kilojoules, fats and proteins.

See also CALCIUM, CARBOHYDRATES, IRON, NUTRIENTS IN FOOD, PROTEIN, SOY PRODUCTS and VITAMINS.

ATTENTION DEFICIT HYPERACTIVITY DISORDER (ADHD)

ADHD is characterised as persistent and age-inappropriate difficulties, particularly lack of attention and hyperactivity–impulsivity, or both. It affects about 5 per cent of young children, although some research indicates it may affect as many as 20 per cent of school-age children to some degree. It accounts for most of the problems seen in kids with special educational needs. ADHD behavioural patterns start at about three to five years of age and the condition affects three times more boys than girls. ADHD can be a chronic lifetime disorder and will continue to affect about 70 per cent of sufferers into their adulthood.

A family history of behavioural or psychiatric disorders is common among children with ADHD, although no specific gene has yet been identified. Increasing amounts of environmental toxins, genetic predisposition and the change in our food are all factors that have been associated with ADHD. Abnormalities in the body's fatty acid metabolism are also closely linked to this disorder.

There is mounting evidence that inadequate amounts of unsaturated fatty acids (omega 3 and 6) have a key role in behavioural and mental problems. Unsaturated fatty acids are crucial for brain development, structure and proper functioning. (Males are thought to be more vulnerable to ADHD, as oestrogen helps females conserve fatty acids, and testosterone may inhibit synthesis of fats.) Omega 3 fatty acids are continually being researched and trialled, with promising results turning up. Randomised controlled trials have shown that unsaturated fatty acids can reduce behavioural and learning difficulties in those with ADHD.

Eighty to 90 per cent of children with ADHD receive some form of medication. Stimulants, not sedatives, are usually prescribed, and 20 to 35 per cent of children don't respond well. These drugs come with many side effects and, moreover, their long-term safety and effectiveness are not known. There is great concern about whether the drugs create a dependency or addictive behaviour when these kids grow up.

Helpful foods

- oily fish such as sustainably caught cod, mackerel, sardines and anchovies
- flaxseed oil, chia seeds and walnuts for their omega 3 properties
- olive oil for its unsaturated fatty acids
- grains such as spelt, kamut, brown rice, barley, millet, amaranth, rye and oats, and seeds such as quinoa

- organic goats milk products—they are anti-inflammatory and easier to digest than cows milk
- tahini, a great source of unsaturated fat and a good source of calcium and essential fatty acids
- organic soy, almond, oat, quinoa or rice milk instead of cows milk
- nut butters, good alternatives to peanut butter, for their good oils
- hummus for its plant protein and good oils
- avocado for its monounsaturated fat
- those high in zinc, magnesium and B vitamins, as they are needed for fatty acid metabolism (see *Nutrients in food*).

Foods to avoid

- food colourings, flavours and all preservatives—the worst ones of this bad bunch are tartrazine (102-yellow) and carmoisine (120-red)
- refined sugar
- refined wheat products, such as bread, pasta, cakes, biscuits, muffins, pizza, crackers, pies, donuts and noodles
- baker's yeast—it contains more acid than you realise
- cow and sheep dairy products, especially if they're conventionally produced
- processed and refined oils and fats, including trans fats
- soft drinks, with or without sugar
- undiluted fruit juices, as they are too concentrated—fresh fruit is okay as it still contains the fibre that slows down the absorption of fructose (sugar)
- refined, processed and packaged foods
- large fish such as swordfish—they have been found to contain unsafe levels of mercury
- fried foods
- artificial sweeteners.

Herbal medicine

- *Ginkgo biloba* helps the brain to store, hold and retrieve information and also sharpens memory
- panax and ginseng improve mental performance—taking ginkgo and panax together has been shown to be more effective than taking them separately
- bacopa for concentration, processing information and mental reactions
- valerian to help with sleep—a good night's sleep leads to improved daytime behaviour
- pine bark extract is likely to be helpful, as it is a great antioxidant
- if you're on medication you will need to take liver herbs such as dandelion root, schisandra or St Mary's thistle to help detox your body of its side effects.

Supplements

- EPA fatty acids (see page 335) from evening primrose oil and flaxseed
- essential fatty acids from vitamin E
- thyme essential oil—simply put a few drops in the bath or oil burner.

Lifestyle factors

- get adequate rest and sleep—ADHD children commonly have sleep disorders
- check for lead toxicity and other heavy metal and chemical toxicity, and deal with any underlying disorders
- ADHD children are likely to have an atopic gene (see *Inflammatory conditions*), and this gene and diabetes interfere with fat metabolism, so avoid obesity and other conditions that may lead to diabetes
- avoid caffeine, alcohol and stress, as these interfere with fat metabolism
- also consider homoeopathy treatments from a reputable practitioner
- avoid canned foods and plastics, as they usually contain BPAs and thalites

🎋 avoid using a microwave

🎋 use only natural, preferably organic, cleaning and body products so your home is chemical-free

🎋 restrict time spent on the computer and smart phones and on watching TV in favour of spending more time exercising outside

🎋 encourage chewing—mindful eating is very important (and apparently difficult for those on ADHD drugs)

🎋 consider a form of exercise that encourages focus—perhaps a martial art, tap dancing or swimming.

See also MEMORY, NUTRIENTS IN FOOD, OILS, SLEEP, VITAMINS and ZINC.

AUTUMN

Autumn is traditionally a time for harvest. It is a time when the energy in your body moves inwards and downwards, in preparation for winter. The emphasis now needs to be on nurturing, building and supporting your organs for the cold change ahead. It is time to clear the heat of summer from your body.

The wind at this time of year will affect your lungs, making breathing more difficult and coughs more frequent. Traditional Chinese medicine (TCM) believes that wind is the root of many diseases. But wind also has the ability to move the internal blockages that cause emotional outbursts. Healthy lungs will help you maintain your purpose and fulfill arrangements and commitments.

The colon, which is the lung's partner in TCM, is responsible for how well you can 'let go' or 'hold on' in certain situations. In this way, you can see how interconnected your body, mind and spirit are—it is difficult to have or maintain good mental or spiritual health if your bodily organs aren't performing as they should, and vice versa. This is a good time of the year to get rid of any unwanted clothes, unpack boxes or just get rid of things (on any level) you don't need. You will feel better for 'letting go'.

It is likely you will feel run down and tired after you've been sick. This is due to deficient energy in the lungs. Constipation is also likely, due to the relationship between the organs. To strengthen the lungs, use cooking methods such as steaming and boiling. In autumn it is a good idea to eat foods that build your immunity.

Although the organs that need most attention during autumn are the lungs and colon, the liver and gallbladder also need attention, as in TCM these organs are related. Take extra care at this time, as it is easy to suffer from gastrointestinal and respiratory complaints.

Many of us also suffer from *dryness* in autumn—symptoms of this are a dry cough, dry lips, wrinkles, itchiness and constipation. To relieve the symptoms of dryness, you are encouraged to eat *moistening foods*, such as those listed below.

A pungent flavour is important for the lungs at any time of the year, but especially useful during autumn, as this is when your lungs are at their most vulnerable. Depending on your condition, heating or cooling pungents will be needed, as mentioned below in 'For specific ailments'.

> For a persistent cough, which is worse at night, hard to get rid of, makes you thirsty and is often accompanied by a sore throat, try foods that 'nourish and moisten'. See below.

Helpful foods

- apples, pears, persimmons, lima beans, spearmint, peppermint, sweet potato, zucchini, carrots, figs, adzuki beans, grapes, olives, spelt, kamut or rye sourdough bread, millet and brown rice, sustainably caught seafood, soups, leeks, vinegar, yoghurt, lemons, limes, grapefruit, cabbage and fresh nuts

- increase the amount of good oils you eat during autumn, as these will protect your skin and therefore protect your lungs—according to TCM, the condition of your skin reflects the condition of your lungs, perhaps because the skin is your largest organ.
- clams, eggs, lemons and sweet potatoes are sour-flavoured foods that protect the skin from the wind
- oranges, pears, peaches, organic soy products, oysters, clams, green beans, royal jelly (check for allergy) and shiitake mushrooms are foods that build immunity
- figs, pears, pumpkins, parsnips, potato and beetroot are foods that build up blood levels and nourish your blood in time for winter
- when you are sick, fresh ginger helps rid your body of any illness through sweat; and when you are well, dried ginger builds immunity; spicy food, however, should be avoided if you are getting sick often, as it reduces immunity through inducing sweat and causing dryness
- organic soy products (tempeh, miso, soymilk and tofu), vegetables (mushrooms, spinach and locally sourced sea vegetables), fruit (apples, pears and persimmons), nuts (almonds, peanuts and pine nuts), grains (barley and millet) and sesame seeds are moistening foods.

Foods to avoid

- cold drinks and ice, melons, salads and raw foods, juices, raw onions, dried spices and chillies
- quick cooking methods such as stir-frying.

For specific ailments

- Low immunity: try leek and garlic soup
- First day of a cold: spring onion, ginger and mint soup

- Arthritis, slow movements, diarrhoea and heavy abdomen: green tea, mushrooms, fennel, cayenne, garlic, onions and ginger
- Run down: bok choy with ginger or garlic
- Cough: foods that 'nourish and moisten'
- Yellow or green (hot) phlegm: use cooling pungents, such as peppermint, chamomile, daikon, radish, watercress and locally sourced sea vegetables
- White (cool) phlegm: use warming pungents, such as garlic, onion, horseradish and ginger
- For either coloured phlegm: use potato, pumpkin, tuna, turnip and mushrooms.

Lifestyle factors

- cook at lower temperatures for longer times, using more water—stews, casseroles and soups during autumn
- this is a time to study and plan
- keep warm
- unresolved grief associated with the lungs and colon will manifest as bronchitis or asthma, or malfunctions of the colon, so it is important to address any underlying feelings of grief or sadness to keep the energy flowing freely through your lungs. If energy or qi is blocked in your lungs, it is difficult to receive energy from the air and the food you eat into your lungs, making it harder for your immunity to ward off illness.

See also ASTHMA, COLDS AND 'FLU, ENERGY, IMMUNITY and TASTE.

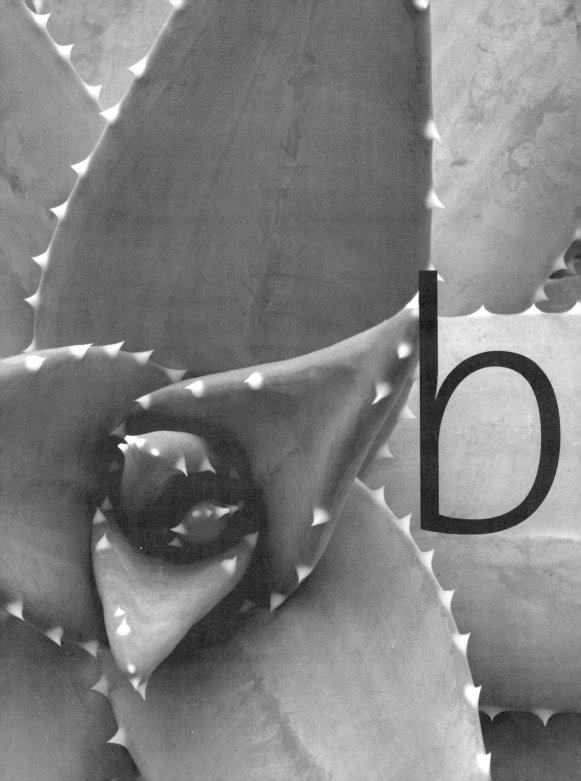

BABY, NUTRITION

Considering your baby's nutritional requirements from the day of birth (or, even better, *in utero*) is one of the wisest parenting decisions you will make. Poor choices will adversely affect a child's health throughout his life. I recommend you exclusively breastfeed your baby until he is at least six months old, although twelve months would be better but not always possible or desirable. The first solids you give your baby will determine what he craves later in life, so it is a good idea to avoid sugar, salt and oily foods. Teaching him early in life by example shows him how a particular food affects his mood and behaviour and helps him to make his own commonsense choices as he grows.

Helpful foods

☙ At **four to six** months start introducing puréed vegetables—Japanese pumpkin first, then sweet potato and carrots. Fruit such as red apples, bananas and pears are also fine. Puréed sweet potato and apple is a lovely combination that freezes well in an ice cube container and may be served with a cereal (as below) or as a dessert with goats yoghurt. With regards to rice, quinoa, amaranth or millet cereal, use a soft organic one, but you should really wait until the baby is at least six months old, when his digestive system can cope with it, before serving this. You can then mix the rice cereal with bancha tea or the liquid from soaked chia seeds, for their calcium, or use breast or goats milk.[1]

---

1   Goats milk is a far better choice than cows milk, as it is very similar to our own milk and easy to digest due to its smaller fat globules. It can be introduced to a breastfed baby around the age of six to eight months, or any time after birth if you are not breastfeeding for whatever reason. Goats milk has about ten times the amount of fluorine than cows milk, which is important for immunity, teeth and bones. Fresh goats milk is best but it will last only seven days in the refrigerator, although it freezes well. Cows milk can make your baby prone to food allergies and diabetes—it is for those with strong digestive tracts and, as baby's tracts aren't mature, it is advisable to avoid it.

Babies also love the texture of jelly squares made from fresh fruit juice, bancha tea and agar agar (see *Sea vegetables*). At this age, it's not so much about taste as about the texture of the food. The water from the soaked chia seed will also set things in almost the same way as agar agar. And they are high in fibre and omega 3 oils. Avocado may be introduced here as well.

- At **six to eight** months puréed green peas and beans can be added to your baby's diet. If you want to give your child animal products, chicken or turkey broth may be introduced. Please buy organic produce, as his little immune system isn't fully developed yet, so he can't deal with the hormones and antibiotics used in non-organic farming. Oats and spelt flakes may also be added now.

- At **eight to twelve** months dark green vegetables, such as zucchini and broccoli, and red vegetables, such as capsicum and tomato, can be given, but not before eight months. Beetroot, turnips and spinach should be introduced last due to their high nitrate content, which is a difficult substance for a baby's body to deal with. Apricots may be introduced at around eight months, but other stone fruit, such as nectarines and prunes, should be left until ten months. Citrus can also be given at ten months. Green apples shouldn't be introduced until around twelve months, as they are too acidic. Rockmelon, honeydew and watermelon can't be introduced until around twelve months because a mould on the skin of these fruits, which may be harmful to a baby, is transferred onto the fruit when it is cut. It is best if all foods are cooked and puréed, and breast milk should still comprise about 50 per cent of baby's diet. Other foods that can be introduced at this age are:
  - low-starch vegetables, which are best
  - vegetable juices are good, especially carrot
  - eggs are okay in moderation from twelve months on—organic ones, please

- organic soy products such as tempeh (best), soymilk and tofu are also recommended
- fruit juices are too concentrated for consumption at this age, so serve them sparingly, as they will weaken your baby's digestion and create a dependency on sugar
- sprouts are low in complex carbohydrates, making them a good choice
- a small amount of locally sourced sea vegetables is wonderful (see *Sea vegetables*)
- fish may also be introduced around twelve months but it should be sustainably caught; avoid tuna or farmed fish.

🐾 Around **eighteen months** the first molar teeth will appear, suggesting that baby's stomach juices are getting ready for more solid food; however, the majority of the diet should still come from grains, cereals and vegetables. Now is the time to slowly introduce legumes such as split peas and starchy vegetables. Be sure to soak the legumes overnight before cooking.

🐾 After about **two years** of age you can introduce more protein and carbohydrates, as baby's digestive tract has matured. It isn't advisable to introduce these foods until now as they need to be chewed properly and a child under the age of two isn't able to do this.

Foods to avoid

🐾 sugar or sweeteners of any kind; your child will find these soon enough

🐾 salty and oily foods

🐾 too much garlic, spices, soy sauces and other strong flavours

🐾 cows milk before twelve months of age. If you must use cows milk, be sure it is organic and raw, and include homogenised—a quick boil will destroy any bacteria or harmful microbes that may be present (boiling also helps to break down its proteins, making it somewhat easier to digest and decreasing potential allergic reactions)—and serve it separately from other food; never serve it cold

- avoid formulas—if you must use one, then choose one with a goats milk base, but some children react to processing of any type
- animal protein until two years old (apart from goats milk products)—if you are really uncomfortable with this, then give them organic chicken, fish or meat broth in moderation.

Lifestyle factors

- don't bribe your child with sweets, or they will link sweets with emotional rather than physical nourishment
- teach them to chew or at least leave their food in their mouths and let it partially dissolve in saliva
- avoid arguments at the dinner table
- eat at the table with the whole family—watching TV while eating teaches them very bad habits
- don't force your child to eat something they don't like—try some other tactic—and don't force them to eat when they are tired, sick or over-excited
- as they have small stomachs, it is better to give your child nourishing snacks if they have missed a meal, rather than forcing large meals on them
- encourage your children to help you in the kitchen—make this an enjoyable time, not a chore
- try not to be too forceful with what you give them, even if you think it's good for them, as kids are prone to losing their appetite from time to time—allow this to pass, supplementing with nutritious snack food
- Smoothies are a brilliant way to get nutrients into the fussy eater, or just when their appetite is low. Use coconut water or another milk as a base, then add flax or coconut oil, chia seeds, LSA, raw cacao

powder and any micro-nutrient you have, such as spirulina, barley or wheatgrass. Add some fruit such as paw paw or berries.

See also Bancha tea; Children, nutrition; Kids' lunchboxes; Lactation; Mastitis; Nutrients in food; and Sea vegetables.

BANCHA TEA

Bancha (*ban* meaning 'number' and *cha* meaning 'tea') is also referred to as Sannen Bancha ('third year bancha'), as it is harvested in the third year of the green tea plant. It is made from the twigs of the plant, not the leaves, therefore you may also see it called 'Twig Tea' or 'Kukicha'. It contains very little, if any, caffeine, so it is suitable for children. Bancha stimulates digestion and is wonderful if you suffer from period pain. It also improves your circulation and warms your body.

To make, pour boiling water over bancha twigs and add one teaspoon of sliced fresh ginger. This is a lovely tea for all year round, as bancha is a spleen tonic, so it helps produce red blood cells—great for building up iron levels. A wonderful circulatory stimulant during winter, the ginger is antioxidant and reduces inflammation. Bancha has about four times more calcium than cows milk.

Try sweetening bancha tea by adding some raw honey or rice syrup, or an umeboshi plum with the ginger for improved digestion. Mix the tea with agar agar that has been dissolved in fruit or vegetable juice, then pour it into ice cube trays and let it set in the fridge—a lovely recipe for babies six months or over.

See also Herbal teas.

BARLEY

Whole barley is more nutritious than pearled barley, has more fibre, twice the calcium, three times the iron and 25 per cent more protein. It builds the blood, benefits the gall bladder and nerves and is easy to digest. Roasted barley is a great coffee substitute; roasting alkalises the barley and aids digestion. It also helps infants tolerate mother's milk. Available as a flour or grain, it contains gluten.

See also WHOLEGRAINS.

BEE POLLEN

Refer to ROYAL JELLY AND BEE POLLEN.

BLOOD SUGAR

To avoid falling victim to the ever-increasing incidence of adult-onset diabetes (type 2), you are urged to reduce foods with a high glycaemic index (GI) because of the way these foods are absorbed by your body. Highly refined or processed foods (those with high GI) dramatically increase blood sugar levels, leaving you feeling elated and full of energy—momentarily. The problem is that what goes up must come down. And the faster it goes up, the faster it comes down. The result of this sudden fall is commonly referred to as 'crashing'. Those who have experienced symptoms of hypoglycaemia (low blood sugar) will tell you it's not pleasant—they include feeling faint, irritable, vague and anxious, with a strong craving for sugar, refined carbs and/or caffeine. If the seesaw action of highs and lows persists, what you eventually develop is diabetes.

The foods that cause your blood sugar to drastically increase are refined sugars and carbohydrates—that is, milk chocolate, white flour and sugar. If it is used to increase energy, coffee should also be avoided, as it exhausts your adrenal glands, which can lead to illnesses such as chronic fatigue and syndrome X—not to mention those unsightly black circles under your eyes.

Foods with sugars that are slower to absorb (low GI foods) are more desirable as they don't lead to sudden bursts and crashes. These foods include complex carbohydrates such as wholegrains, fruit, vegetables, legumes, nuts and seeds.

See also BREAD, CARBOHYDRATES and DIABETES, TYPE 2.

BREAD

Bread has changed so much over the past 50 years that it no longer contains the amount of vitamins and minerals it once did. Many would argue that packaged white flour has no nutritional value at all—it is simply used as a medium for toppings such as jam, butter, cheese and meats. Bread was once a flavoursome, nutritious and sharing food in its own right. Real bread is made using freshly ground flour, leaven (a substance that produces fermentation) and a wood-fired oven—that's it, nothing artificial added. If you haven't tasted this type of bread, you don't know what you're missing. The 1950s saw a demise in regional bakers and more and more commercial bakeries started adding a variety of substances, such as malt compounds, glycerine, 'improvers' and chemical shortenings. The grain was also modified so that it contained three to four times the amount of gluten. This was apparently due to the general feeling that brown or wholemeal bread was somehow inferior, only suitable for the poorest of people. And remember, gluten translates to 'glue' in Latin. Isn't that how you feel after you've eaten white bread?

The health problems that have arisen from this type of commercially produced bread are numerous and varied—people complain of nausea, bloating, fatigue, skin problems, asthma and other allergies, abdominal cramping, indigestion, reflux, diarrhoea, constipation, or a combination of these symptoms, plus many more. Our bodies just don't recognise the current wheat grain as a food, therefore they reject it. Grains used be much larger and contained a higher amount of protein and fibre.

Flavourless, colourless and devoid of nutrients, bread in its current form has no place in a healthy diet. Even wholemeal bread is not much better than white, as it is usually artificially coloured to make it look brown, then nutrients are added to try and replace what has been lost during the manufacturing. It doesn't. The bran and germ of bleached flour have been removed and a range of chemicals added. Bleaching, which destroys most of the flour's nutrients, also acts chemically to age and soften flour as well as repel insects.

Most countries in Europe do not permit flour to be adulterated at all. Australia, sadly, has no such laws. Britain requires that the nutrients lost during bleaching and sifting be artificially replaced. This seems like a waste of time and energy and again doesn't really replace what has been lost nutritionally or in taste.

Yeast is a relatively recent addition to bread—it was discovered in a French chemist's lab 100 years ago. The problem with yeast is that using it requires the addition of a lot more salt. If you make bread at home and want to use yeast, try to use compressed yeast, which keeps in the fridge. Dried yeast may produce a strong rise and crumbly bread, but in general, you need to use twice as much dried yeast as compressed yeast. It interferes with the balance of bacteria in your gut.

Many people have enormous trouble digesting gluten—the protein in wheat, oats, barley and rye—especially if it is added. Adding gluten flour to bread is a way to make the loaf spring back if it is compressed but it is a fraudulent bread-making technique. Some wholegrains containing gluten are easier to digest because they are 'whole' grains, but it is still best to seek out 'real' bread.

These are the original grains and methods of bread-making that haven't been tampered with:

100 per cent rye (schwartzbrot) This bread lends itself beautifully to accompaniments such as dill pickles and sustainably caught fish. Caraway, dill or cumin seeds make the rye more digestible.

Essene breads These easily digested breads are made by using crushed five-day-old wheat sprouts. They are very high in enzymes, and taste and look somewhat like pumpernickel—dark, slightly sour and moist.

Kamut This unadulterated older cereal variety from ancient Egypt has grains that are often three times the size of wheat. It is high in protein as well as being rich in amino acids and vitamins. It is easy to digest.

Sourdough This is the name given to naturally risen bread with no added bakers' yeast; instead a sourdough culture, which can be hundreds of years old, is used. It is the most ancient technique used to leaven bread and it is still in everyday use in Europe and gaining popularity in Australia. Furthermore, this natural-rise starter has significant health benefits—it is high in B vitamins, especially B12; the calcium is also more easily absorbed by your body; it helps to generate good intestinal flora, thus aiding digestion; and it is more nutritious five to ten days after baking. Using this type of leaven makes wheat more digestible.

Spelt This original wheat grain from Persia contains gluten, but is easily digested by most people. It contains seven of the eight essential amino acids and is an ideal substitute for wheat flour.

Stone-ground flour The grains for the flour are crushed by two circular stones, a method that makes bread superior in taste to roller-milled flour. All flour was stoneground until the nineteenth century.

Wholemeal flour This type of flour contains all the original components of the wheat grain as long as it is the 'real' type, not the stuff bought off supermarket shelves.

See also BLOOD SUGAR, CARBOHYDRATES and DIABETES, TYPE 2.

BRONCHITIS
Refer to ASTHMA, AUTUMN and IMMUNITY.

BUCKWHEAT
Buckwheat, despite its name, is not a cereal (grass). It is a plant native to central Asia and its seeds are ground into a flour. This flour is used to make soba noodles, blini and breads and cakes. Buckwheat contains the

bioflavonoid rutin, which is wonderful for treating conditions that lead to heart problems, such as poor circulation and high blood pressure, by strengthening capillaries and blood vessels. Sprouted buckwheat is high in chlorophyll, enzymes and vitamins and, after roasting, it is an alkaline-forming food. Insects don't find it appealing, so it is grown without the use of chemicals—actually buckwheat will die if it is sprayed.

Sprouted buckwheat is a great source of enzymes, chlorophyll and vitamins. It improves appetite and strengthens digestion. Gluten-free, it is available as a grain, flour, pasta or noodle (udon or soba)—look for 100 per cent buckwheat, otherwise refined wheat flour will usually be added.

See also CARDIOVASCULAR HEALTH, STRESS and WHOLEGRAINS.

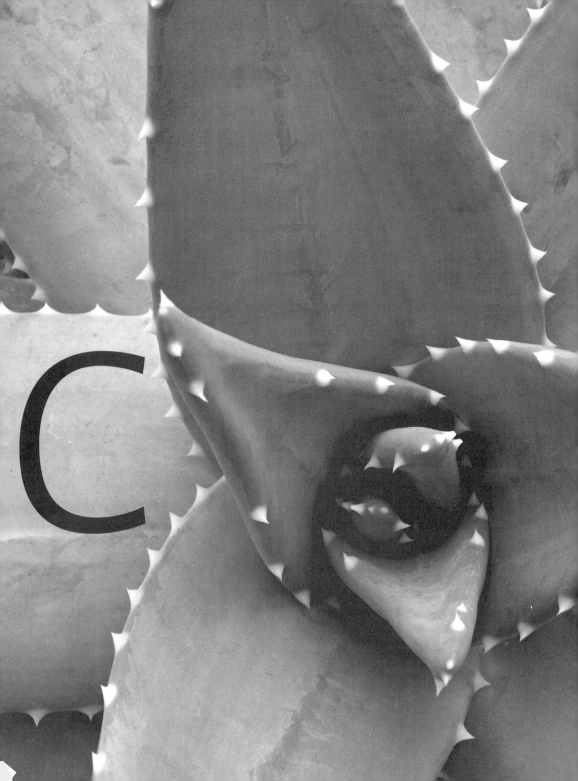

CACAO

Cacao, pronounced ka-cow, better known to us in the past as cocoa, has been gaining quite a reputation over the last few years. How did we get it so wrong—adding sugar, milk powder caramels and other unnecessary additives to this wonderfully giving bean to make an inferior product?

Once used as currency in Mexico, cacao was worshipped as a sacred food by the ancient Mayan and Aztec cultures. The Latin name for the cacao tree—*Theobroma cacao*—means food of the gods. Modern science has now confirmed that raw cacao is the most nutritionally complex food on the planet.

It contains super high levels of antioxidants—while blueberries contain 32 antioxidants and wild blueberries 61, cacao beans contain an unbelievable 621. The powder is considered a 'raw' food, with all its heat-sensitive vitamins, minerals and antioxidants remaining intact, thereby maximising digestion and absorption. Raw cacao products are also a source of beta-carotene, amino acids (protein), omega 3 EFAs, calcium, vitamin C, zinc, iron, copper, sulfur, potassium and one of the best food sources of muscle relaxing—stress-relieving magnesium.

Recently we have been learning of its wonderful affect on the cardio-vascular system, especially for lowering blood pressure. It's also a great source of fibre and helps to keep your blood sugar balanced.

Add the powder to your smoothies, truffles, desserts and sauces. Never again do you have to feel guilty about eating chocolate, but just make sure it's raw and dark.

CALCIUM

In the Western world we have a high intake of cows dairy and a high incidence of osteoporosis, so perhaps we need alternative sources of calcium that contain magnesium to help the calcium get into the bones, and without all the additives that cows milk contains.

It has been shown that animal protein causes the body to excrete calcium more quickly than plant protein. Coffee also has this effect, along with an excess of unfermented soy products such as milk and tofu. Rich sources of calcium include leafy green vegetables, dried fruit, nuts and seeds (including chia seeds), molasses, locally sourced sea vegetables and tahini. Parsley and other herbs are also good sources.

Green plants are higher in calcium than any other food. However, beet greens, plums, cranberry, silver beet and unhulled tahini are high in oxalic acid, which inhibits calcium absorption.

Calcium is essential for the proper functioning of your heart, bones, nerves and muscles. It is necessary for:

- the prevention of cardiovascular disease
- muscle growth and the prevention of cramps
- blood clotting
- strong bones, teeth and gums
- the prevention of cancer and osteoporosis
- energy
- the breakdown of fats
- healthy skin
- proper digestion
- the nervous system.

Recommended daily intake of calcium

Stage of life	RDI (mg per day)
	Females
Up to 7 years	800
8–11 years	900
12–15 years	1000
16–54 years	800
Post-menopausal	1000
Pregnant—first two trimesters	1100
Pregnant—last trimester and lactating	1200

Stage of life	RDI (mg per day)
	Males
Up to 11 years	800
12–15 years	1200
16–18 years	1000
19 years and over	800

Calcium is essential for the proper functioning of your heart, bones, nerves and muscles. Calcium uptake depends on the health of your kidney/adrenal function. When calcium is deficient, all other minerals will be out of whack. Without magnesium, phosphorus and vitamins A, C and D in your diet, calcium won't be absorbed. Magnesium is essential for pulling calcium into your bones.

Signs of calcium deficiency include:

- depression, anxiety and panic attacks
- delusions, convulsions and hyperactivity
- heart palpitations, high cholesterol and blood pressure
- tooth decay, aching joints and brittle nails
- poor bone density
- eczema and arthritis.

There are times when calcium requirements increase. These include:

- older age, especially for women
- when you have bone or teeth and gum problems
- when suffering from heart conditions
- during periods of stress
- at times of growth—pregnancy and lactation, childhood and adolescence
- when digestion is poor
- when you undertake regular, excessive exercise.

Age, menopause in women and poor digestion are common reasons for calcium deficiency. Caucasian women are eight times more likely to develop osteoporosis, a disease due to calcium loss, than Caucasian men.

Calcium-rich foods	Milligrams per 1000 mg food
Agar agar	400
Almonds	233
Chia seeds	500
Chicken	11
Chickpeas	150
Cows milk	119
Cows yoghurt	121
Ground beef	10
Hazelnuts	209
Kelp	1099
Nori	260
Parsley	203
Quinoa	141
Salmon	79
Sardines	443
Sesame seeds	110
Sunflower seeds	174
Tempeh	93
Tofu, firm	100
Watercress	151
Wheatgrass and barley grass (dried)	514

Helpful foods

- leafy green vegetables, such as kale, rocket, English spinach, Asian greens and watercress; green plants are higher in calcium than any other food
- grains, such as brown rice, barley, quinoa, oats and millet
- legumes, such as chickpeas and mung, lima and soybeans
- locally sourced sea vegetables, such as nori and kelp
- dried fruit, nuts, seeds (especially chia seeds) and molasses
- tahini
- parsley
- fermented dairy (easiest to digest), including yoghurt, quark and kefir

- alfalfa
- silicon-rich foods (silicon increases calcium absorption), including celery, lettuce, parsnips, oats, brown rice, strawberries, cucumber, apricots and carrots
- foods high in lysine (for calcium absorption)—eggs, sustainably caught fish, lima beans and organic soy products
- magnesium-rich foods
- chia seeds.

Foods to avoid

- beet greens, plums and cranberry, which are high in oxalic acid, limiting calcium absorption
- too many sweet foods, as they interfere with calcium absorption, causing bone loss and osteoarthritis
- too much protein, especially from meat
- too much salt
- refined flour (white), sugar (white), any sweeteners and salt
- too much or too little exercise
- Nightshade family of vegetables, such as tomatoes, potatoes, eggplant, capsicum and chillies
- coffee, cigarettes, alcohol and marijuana
- junk food of all kinds.

Herbal medicine

- dried horsetail as a tea; it is high in silicon
- medicinal herbs, such as alfalfa, chamomile, fennel seed, lemongrass, nettle (really high in iron and calcium), parsley, paprika, peppermint, red clover, rosehip and yarrow
- culinary herbs to use are alfalfa, fennel seed, lemongrass, parsley and paprika.

Lifestyle factors

- exercise moderately and regularly
- get some sun—vitamin D helps to utilise calcium.

See also ARTHRITIS, CANCER, CARDIOVASCULAR HEALTH, DIGESTION, ENERGY, MAGNESIUM, MENOPAUSE, OSTEOPOROSIS and TEETH AND GUM PROBLEMS.

CANCER

At last diet has been linked to degenerative diseases, including some cancers, through a number of studies. It seems logical that with a diet free of processed and refined grains and oils, along with a reduction in exposure to free radicals, you greatly reduce your chance of getting cancer, but it has taken a while for proof to appear. To maximise your protection against cancer, reduce—if not eliminate—red meat, dairy, sugar, hydrogenated vegetable oils and added chemicals, hormones and antibiotics in food from your diet.

Other factors that add to the high incidence of cancers in our society are the depletion of minerals from our soils, less home cooking, a sedentary lifestyle, overeating (especially of rich foods) and radiation fallout from TV sets, irradiated foods from overseas, toxic cleaning and body products, mobile phones, computer monitors, microwaves, X-rays and powerlines. Decreased immunity, as always, is also implicated, as are environmental toxins from cars, industry and factory farming . . . the list goes on. No wonder organic produce is gaining in popularity, and rightly so. When treating or preventing cancers, the entire human organism needs to be addressed, especially the liver. Oxygen deficiency or starvation has been said to be the greatest cause of all disease.

Anyone can follow the guidelines below, especially if there is a strong genetic predisposition towards cancer.

Helpful foods

- juices of leafy dark green vegetables and sprouts in large doses—about two to six glasses a day consumed at room temperature (be sure to drink them separately from meals, otherwise they may cause fermentation in your gut). Recommended juices are carrot, beetroot (the roots and tops of which cleanse the liver and blood and lubricate the intestines, so they are useful for reducing constipation), parsley, celery, kale, cabbage, capsicum, sprouts, wheatgrass and garlic
- foods high in betacarotene—such as orange, yellow, red and green fruits and vegetables—convert to vitamin A in the body, which protects against cancer
- kale has more antioxidants than any other veggie. Add it to your smoothies, and eat lots of it. To get the most out of kale, cook it a little
- potatoes are high in potassium, which is needed to combat cancers
- onions and garlic are anti-cancer agents due to their high content of quercetin—one onion a day is recommended for inhibiting cellular growth while garlic reduces associated yeast infections (if you can manage to eat raw garlic, chew half a clove twice a day or add it to your juice; to freshen your breath, chew on some raw parsley)
- daikon (white radish) helps to cleanse toxic residue from animal products that feed cancers and tumours; it 'cools' your liver
- asparagus, great for detoxing, is a diuretic (removes excess water) and able to increase circulation through its high content of vitamin E
- the Brassica family of vegetables—including cauliflower, broccoli, brussels sprouts and cabbage—has anti-cancer and antioxidant properties; these vegetables stimulate liver function, and contain sulfur, which is antibiotic and antiviral
- mushrooms—particularly the Japanese mushrooms, reishi, maitake and shiitake—have the ability to neutralise the toxic residue from animal

products, which increases oxygenation in the body (these mushrooms are now available as a supplement, as they have potential anti-tumour properties—they are said to contain interferon, a protein that may stimulate an immune response against cancers and viruses)

- corn is known to stimulate metabolism and increase oxygenation
- butyrate, formed from the fibre in wholegrains, suppresses cancer—alkaline-forming grains such as millet and roasted buckwheat are the best choices; amaranth is also recommended, but quinoa is best eaten in moderation, as it is high in protein and fat. All grains must be chewed properly to aid digestion and thus absorption
- turmeric is a good anti-inflammatory and liver tonic; juice it, add it to your meals and smoothies
- watercress may reduce cancerous growths
- omega 3 oils from flaxseed, chia seeds, walnuts, leafy dark green vegetables and pumpkin seeds
- vitamin E-rich foods fight cancer
- paw paw is great, as it breaks down undigested animal meat, destroys parasites and dries up the internal 'dampness' often associated with cancers
- grape, mango, cherry, pomegranate, radish and cranberry are beneficial
- oats have long been recommended to cancer patients—they are high in B vitamins, so they relax your nervous system; their fibre will cleanse your arteries and reduce mucus in your body; their mucilaginous properties will soothe inflamed digestive tracts
- rye is another grain to include as it dries 'dampness'—if you eat it as sourdough bread it is much easier to digest
- sprouts of legumes, especially mung and adzuki.

Foods to avoid

- cucumbers, as they promote the right environment for cancers
- melons, pineapples, pears, peaches, fresh figs and citrus fruit, as they are too watery and may contribute to cancerous growths
- coconut and avocados, as they are too fatty (of course a little is okay); coconut water, however, is recommended
- dried fruit, as it is too sweet—apart from dried figs, which are okay
- berries and plums, as they are too acidic
- soy products as, due to their high protein content, they promote tumour growth—don't completely eliminate, only reduce
- white sugar can cause tumours and growths to spread
- yeasted breads
- processed and refined grains and oils
- animal products, including dairy and red meat. Fish that is high in omega 3 oils may be included if there is severe weakness; goats milk products are mostly tolerated
- wheat, as it promotes tissue growth and may cause allergies—if sweating or insomnia is present then grains such as spelt or kamut and essene (sprouted-grain) breads may be useful
- sweet foods, including fruit, promote dampness in the body
- salt decreases potassium (mostly provided by potatoes and fruit and vegetables in general) in the body, which is vital when fighting cancer—salt should not be added to the diet, but should come from locally sourced sea vegetables and herbs; also avoid too many salty foods such as miso and soy sauces, especially from Japan
- margarine will increase your risk of cancer and heart disease
- nuts and seeds (apart from flaxseeds and a small amount—six per day—of almonds) are too oily, and thus heavy on your liver—peanuts are a definite no-no, as they contain a carcinogenic compound.

Herbal medicine for the cancer patient

- chaparral is anti-cancerous
- turmeric for the liver and as an antioxidant
- pau d'arco is antifungal and immune-enhancing
- astragalus improves digestion, increases energy and helps with nutrient absorption—it helps hasten recovery after chemotherapy and radiation therapy
- dandelion root is antiviral, antifungal and often used in cancer therapy
- poke root is anti-cancerous—be sure to take only as directed, as it is toxic in large doses
- echinacea enhances immunity and cleans the blood
- grape seed extract, one of the most powerful antioxidants available, will reduce swelling and inflammation
- immune-boosting cat's claw has anti-tumour properties
- astralagus also has anti-tumour properties
- aloe vera gel applied topically will heal any skin disorders associated with radiation.

Supplements

- wheat or barley grass will help detox and stimulate the liver, cool it down and reduce inflammation in the gastrointestinal tract. As they are both high in chlorophyll they will help with cellular oxygenation and promote a healthy intestinal flora. Wheatgrass will also counteract the effects of radiation and combat the effects of chemotherapy
- vitamin C in small doses (500 mg, three to five times a day) is one of the most important supplements generally; during chemotherapy or radiation therapy the dose may increase substantially—vitamin C is an antioxidant that will detoxify blood
- kelp and other sea vegetables are very high in minerals (needed for vitamin and enzyme action), have the ability to soften hardened

masses in the body and are also packed with iodine, which improves thyroid function and oxygenation—avoid if stools are watery. Avoid sea vegetables from Japan

- spirulina and chlorella are high in vitamin A (an antioxidant) and protect cells from damage
- flaxseed oil has anti-tumour properties and is an antioxidant
- GLA oils, found in spirulina and evening primrose oil, are helpful
- royal jelly and bee pollen (check that you're not allergic to these) have anti-cancer qualities—they contain all of the essential nutrients
- coenzyme Q10 improves cellular oxygenation
- B12 supplementation may be necessary if you are on a predominantly vegetarian diet, but only if your digestion isn't working effectively.

Lifestyle factors for cancer treatment

- improve liver health (see *Liver*)
- acupuncture is helpful for reducing stagnant energy in your body
- decrease fermentation in your gut and increase enzyme activity by drinking juices separately from meals and by avoiding stress and the foods in 'Foods to avoid'
- Swedish massage may spread cancer, so avoid—consider a shiatsu massage instead
- See *Sugar alternatives* for ways to satisfy sweet cravings; raw honey may also be used in moderation for this
- when choosing a juicer, be sure to get one that has slow revolutions (ones that juice too quickly heat up the enzymes of the juice, destroying them). You will need to cut the food pieces smaller, but the juice will last up to 72 hours in the fridge and have its enzymes intact; be sure to drink the juices at room temperature
- drink only pure water, definitely not tap water; see *Water* for the best filter to buy

- it is really important not to overeat
- reduce stress by trying to resolve any old, underlying negative emotions
- increase oxygenation by exercising moderately and regularly and eating fresh, light foods
- breathing clean air is important—large cities are full of free radicals (the bad guys); if you haven't done so already, consider a sea or tree move
- eat only whole food; your diet really needs to be fully organic. Avoid denatured, altered or 'changed' foods—those that claim to be 'fat-free', 'low-salt', 'fortified with calcium' etc. and foods using GM technology are definitely out, as are irradiated foods from Europe and any foods from Japan
- your diet should consist of approximately 40 per cent grains, 40 per cent vegetables, 10 per cent fruit, 5 per cent legumes and 5 per cent other—the 'other' could be royal jelly (check for allergy), spirulina or a not-so-naughty treat
- be discerning with the supplements you take—some vitamin pills may aggravate you and/or your gut; less is more
- avoid all caffeine from tea, coffee and soft drinks
- avoid smoking, including passive smoking
- it's really important to avoid as many chemicals as you can—buy natural skin and body care and cleaning products.

See also CANDIDA, FIBRE, FLAXSEEDS, IMMUNITY, OILS, SEA VEGETABLES and VITAMINS.

CANDIDA

For years candida was misdiagnosed or undiagnosed, then it seemed anyone who sought out a health professional was told they had it. Yes, it is very common and, yes, it is extremely taxing on your body, but not everybody has it.

Candida albicans is a naturally occurring yeast-like fungus in the mouth, oesophagus, throat and genital tract. Problems occur when the delicate balance of flora within these regions is disrupted and the immune system of the body weakened. Then the 'bad' bacteria take over and you develop candida, an imbalance in your gut flora.

Most often candida will affect the mouth, ears, nose, gut and vagina. Both men and women are susceptible so it is advisable that both partners are treated as it may be passed through sexual contact. Candida can also affect the whole body. This type of candida is known as *systemic candidiasis* and in extreme cases it can travel through the bloodstream, affecting all your organs. This nasty type of candida is called *Candida septicemia*.

It is quite easy to create an imbalance in the body. Antibiotics have been singled out as the main culprit, but any prescription or recreational drugs (including the contraceptive pill and corticosteroids) as well as pregnancy and AIDS will increase your chances of infection. Of course stress is a major contributor, as are sugar, yeast, junk food and alcohol.

The symptoms include fungal infections such as 'jock itch', tinea (athlete's foot) and some rashes and other skin problems; digestive complaints, such as bloating, nausea, bad breath, malabsorption of nutrients and fatigue; thrush, either vaginal or at the back of your throat; ringworms; fungus under the fingernails or toenails; food intolerances and environmental sensitivities. You might also suffer from memory loss; white spots in the mouth; itchy anus, ears or throat; nappy rash; excess mucus; oedema; a heavy and sluggish feeling; mental dullness; and mood swings.

Helpful foods
- essential fatty acids from sustainably caught fish, flaxseed oil and olive oil will protect your cells from damage
- garlic reduces infection
- yoghurt with live cultures will reduce fungal growth (for maintenance)

- wholefoods, including some sustainably caught fish, organic brown rice, fruit (maximum of one piece a day) and vegetables and legumes (especially mung beans) and other wholegrains
- complex carbohydrates, chewed properly, can be helpful—not harmful as once thought—as they are a good source of lignins, which inhibit the growth of yeast. They are found in high amounts in millet, rye, oats, barley, amaranth, quinoa and roasted buckwheat
- sprouts are wonderful here
- the iodine content of both Australian and New Zealand sea vegetables deactivates yeasts
- green plants—such as kale, parsley, watercress, cabbage, wheatgrass and spirulina—contain high amounts of chlorophyll, which promotes healthy intestinal flora.

Foods to avoid

- sugar, as all forms of candida thrive on it
- yeast, because candida is a yeast and adding baker's yeast just makes the problem a whole lot worse—don't forget yeast is in Vegemite® and Promite® and many other things, so always read the label when buying packaged foods; instead, eat sourdough bread made from spelt, rye or kamut flour
- refined carbohydrates turn very quickly into sugar, on which candida thrives, and aren't usually tolerated by people with this condition anyway; your body will be craving sweet foods, however, so see *Sugar alternatives* for help in this department
- fermented foods, such as tempeh, miso, soy sauce and vinegars— I personally don't think this makes too much difference as, in most cases, cooking them reduces their fermentation. In fact, the stress created by putting someone on a full anti-candida diet often makes the symptoms worse

- fruit, as it is full of fructose (a sugar)—one piece a day should be okay but avoid acidic types, such as oranges, limes, pineapples, grapefruit, lemons and tomatoes; dried fruits are a definite no-no
- nuts and seed, unless freshly roasted.

Herbal medicine

- pau d'arco is an antifungal and antibacterial herb that is immune-boosting—it may be drunk as a tea for maintenance, but you'll need a strong practitioner-only type as well
- thuja is also an antifungal herb
- citrus seed extract is an antimicrobial extract that works in the same way as a fourteen-day antibiotic course—it bombs everything in the gut, good and bad. This is quite a strong treatment so it should be done under the care of a practitioner
- golden seal will help repair inflamed intestinal lining by helping to repair damage to cell membranes
- echinacea is important for boosting immunity, cleaning the blood and as an anti-inflammatory
- clove and pau d'arco tea should be drunk often
- topically, a cream made of pau d'arco, chickweed, neem, golden seal and tea tree is effective.

Supplements

- acidophilus (non-dairy formula) will help balance gut flora. However, try to reduce the candida before taking acidophilus, unless your case is mild, as I have found that giving it before you reduce the overgrowth doesn't make much difference—the bad stuff gobbles it up
- for thrush—eat umeboshi plums or use the diluted vinegar (1:3) as a douche; diluted tea tree oil applied topically or in the bath; a douche of apple cider vinegar and water (1:3); or a douche of pau d'arco

(antifungal) and garlic tea, made by infusing one clove garlic and one tablespoon pau d'arco tea. Leave to cool before using

- inserting a fresh clove of garlic, which has been threaded with cotton, in the vagina and leaving it overnight each night for one week to a month is also very helpful
- apply yoghurt topically to the vagina to reduce fungus growth
- vitamin C for improving immunity; zinc is also helpful.

Lifestyle factors

- try and stay cool—heat and damp environments make it worse (trust me, an Indonesian holiday would be your worst nightmare)
- the sugars in alcohol will exacerbate the condition, and definitely avoid beer—too much sugar and yeast—and an Indonesian holiday
- stress—especially anger, worry and anxiety—really does make it worse
- seek professional advice if you have persistent candida—it may be a symptom of an underlying illness
- check for mercury poisoning, as this can lead to candida
- candida is common in those with HIV/AIDS and also those with a chronic condition on Western medication
- avoid overeating
- reduce consumption of raw foods, as these weaken digestion
- eat simply, avoiding too many flavours in one meal
- it is very important to re-establish good bacteria in the gut after taking antibiotics—use miso, sauerkraut, acidophilus, locally sourced sea vegetables or wheat or barley grass. Remember that animals are fed antibiotics, hormones and a cocktail of other synthetic toxins, so if you are eating animal products, the foods listed in 'Helpful foods' should be a regular part of your diet
- exercise regularly and moderately
- some form of meditation would be of great benefit.

CARBOHYDRATES

Most people feel tired and bloated after a pasta meal or even a salad sandwich. Or they get the 2 p.m. mid-afternoon 'dip' due to too many refined carbohydrates or sugars throughout the morning and at lunch. Yes, these foods fill you up quickly when you're starving or you're on the run, and it's easy to find a place that will serve you refined carbohydrates, such as white rice and bread and pasta. What's not so easy, however, is to find a meal that'll make you feel good after you've eaten it as well as give you useable energy with which to finish the day.

Since the Industrial Revolution wheat has been the staple grain in the West. Our bodies need variety, but many of us are brought up on toast, breakfast cereals, biscuits, crackers, pasta and pastries—all made from wheat—at every meal. Wheat has now been hybridised to the point where the original grain is hardly recognisable. Our current wheat grain is not easily digested, so it causes a variety of symptoms, including weight gain, indigestion, diabetes, cardiovascular complaints, constipation or diarrhoea, hayfever, sinusitis, irritable bowel syndrome, infertility, candida or hypoglycaemia. In addition, coeliac disease rates have risen dramatically.

It's no wonder our digestive tracts have had a 'gutfull'. Refined wheat and its products should be eaten only in moderation, if at all.

As there are so many other grains available to us, it's interesting that processed and refined wheat, closely followed by white rice, has become the principal 'grain' consumed. Complex carbs—grains such as kamut, millet, spelt, quinoa (actually a seed), amaranth, barley and rye are highly nutritious and are often higher in essential minerals, vitamins, complex carbohydrates and protein than animal products. They are mostly in their original form and easily digested, making them preferable food choices. (Complex carbs are also things such as nuts and seeds, legumes and fruit and veggies—not just grains.)

At present low-carb diets are all the rage but they are nothing new. In fact, various health practitioners have been proponents of these since the 1800s. In a time when diseases such as diabetes, multiple sclerosis, cancer and heart disease are on the rise, people are searching for answers—and every food seems to have its day. First, we are told to cut down on fat, then protein (then to increase it), and now carbs are in the firing line.

Most of us consume processed carbohydrates at every meal. These foods, being refined carbohydrates, turn to sugar in your body (even faster if you lead a sedentary lifestyle), which sends your glycaemic index way up while giving you a sugar 'fix'. You may feel momentarily elated after consumption, and perhaps full, but this is closely followed by a terrible 'crash' or low blood sugar.

Insulin, the fat-storing hormone, is stimulated in excess by the pancreas when too many refined carbohydrates and sugars are eaten. If this hormone remains high, due to excessive amounts of carbohydrates in the diet, then ketosis/lipolysis cannot occur. This state is important for weight loss, as it breaks down fat, instead of glucose, to be used as energy by the body and the brain.

Unless it's processed junk food, cutting an entire food group out of your diet is rarely a good idea. Complex carbohydrates are essential for a healthy body and mind. They are loaded with B vitamins, which nourish the nervous system. They provide sustaining long-term energy, proteins for tissue building and fats for lubrication and tissue support. This type of diet is also high in fibre, which allows efficient elimination.

When chewed properly, complex carbohydrates become sweeter, thus diminishing the sweet craving, and make the protein and oils in them more readily available to the body. Complex carbohydrates are also a sharing and nurturing food that (in moderation) makes us feel good. There is no need to cut out carbohydrates altogether, only those that are refined. Retain the complex carbohydrates.

Lifestyle factors

- choose complex carbohydrates instead of the refined ones—slower to be absorbed and higher in essential nutrients, they are whole foods (examples of complex carbohydrates are wholegrains such as quinoa, oats, spelt, brown rice and kamut; legumes, including chickpeas, kidney beans etc.; fruit and vegetables; nuts and seeds)
- eat carbohydrates during the day and less at night—the day is when you need them most; besides, they are high-energy food, and not recommended before sleep
- limit your intake of carbohydrates to 40 to 80 grams per day.

See also BLOOD SUGAR, BREAD and DIABETES, TYPE 2.

CARDIOVASCULAR HEALTH

According to traditional Chinese medicine (TCM), the heart not only regulates the circulation of blood but is also responsible for consciousness, sleep, spirit and memory. It is where the mind is seated. To have good cardiovascular health means you have your heart and mind in balance. If you wonder how emotions affect your heart, then just note how your pulse rate rises when you become anxious or sexually aroused, or notice how someone's health may deteriorate when their heart is broken.

TCM believes that when your shen (spirit) escapes from your heart, it causes a variety of symptoms such as loss of memory, a wandering mind, irrational behaviour, insomnia, irregular heartbeat, confused speech, a weak quivering voice, depression, poor circulation and a ruddy complexion. Foods that help quieten your spirit and help you stay centred are mushrooms; mulberries and lemons; culinary herbs, such as dill and basil; herbal medicine, such as schisandra, dan shen and mandarin; herbal teas, such as chamomile, skullcap and valerian; and goats milk before bedtime.

Happy people will often have healthy hearts. These people are usually humble and open to the wonders of their world. Many of us—traditionally more men than women—deny our true feelings and merely 'soldier on'. This causes us to live more 'in our heads'. You need to remember your heart is your centre, not your brain. The two need to be in balance, however. Denying your true feelings only causes the 'band' around your chest to tighten. This is referred to as 'contraction-band necrosis', and in physical terms it presents itself as angina, atherosclerosis and arteriosclerosis.

The expression 'keeping your cool' means staying cool, calm and collected. In an age where aggression, ambition and an over-analytical mind seem to have become highly respected, we should learn to heed the message behind this expression. It's all about balance and moderation. The 'yang' aspects of modern thoughts and feelings cause your body to overheat, resulting in a worrying mind. Denying the 'yin', or the more creative, feminine, receptive, relaxed, intuitive and creative parts of yourself, exasperates this situation. (Some people refer to the yang and yin as being either predominantly a left- or right-sided brain thinker.)

Numerous studies have now shown us that, on a physical level, good heart health—therefore good heart–mind balance—is related to both calcium and protein metabolism. Some factors that interfere with calcium absorption include coffee, alcohol, marijuana, tobacco, refined flour, salt, refined sugar and pesticides. There is also a direct correlation between high-protein diets and an elevated incidence of heart disease and osteoporosis. The physical symptoms of a heart–mind imbalance are high blood pressure, high cholesterol, arteriosclerosis, atherosclerosis and insomnia.

Finding your soul's purpose, your blueprint, is of vital importance—spiritually, emotionally and physically. True health comes only after the mind, body and spirit are nourished. Instead of thinking about the past or the future, you are encouraged to remain in the 'present' and practise mindfulness. Being 'present' sounds easy enough, but it is seemingly one of the hardest things to do. But this will help you to stay calm, rational, creative and functional. The effect the mind has on your body should not be under-estimated. Controlling your thoughts through disciplined behaviour will have almost immediate, positive results on your health.

Helpful foods

- foods high in vitamin E to improve circulation and blood flow—leafy dark green vegetables, legumes, nuts, seeds, soybeans, wheatgerm and wholegrains (buckwheat and raw cacao have also been used to reduce blood pressure)
- good fats—including olive oil, walnuts, chia seeds, macadamias, flax, avocado, coconut and sustainably caught cold-water fish—may also help in lowering cholesterol
- high-fibre foods—fruit, vegetables, wholegrains, chia seeds, psyllium husks and raw cacao
- garlic, onions and lecithin to lower cholesterol.

Foods to avoid

- processed foods, sugar and flour
- coffee
- soft drinks
- lots of alcohol
- saturated fats (animal fats, such as red meat, milk, cheese and cream)
- milk chocolate
- foods fried in refined oils
- refined salt
- margarine and other trans-fatty acids
- low-fat foods.

Herbal medicine

- hawthorn berries
- globe artichoke
- motherwort
- *Ginkgo biloba.*

Lifestyle factors

- learn a meditation technique—mindfulness helps us to remain present; if you're new to it, get a guide to meditation CD
- maintain a healthy weight
- exercise moderately and regularly
- reduce stress (learn stress management techniques)
- avoid smoking
- monitor blood pressure and cholesterol
- express yourself and your needs
- relax your body
- practise a gentle martial art, such as qi gong or tai qi
- make the necessary changes to enjoy your life
- listen to your higher self.

See also MEMORY, ORGANS AND ASSOCIATED EMOTIONS and SUMMER.

CELLULITE

Cellulite is a term used to describe the dimpled appearance of skin caused by fat deposits that are just below the surface of the skin. It generally appears on skin in the abdomen, lower limbs and pelvic region, and it usually occurs after puberty. Cellulite occurs in both men and women, but it is much more common in women because they are more likely to have particular types of fat and connective tissue.

The causes are not known for sure but it seems these factors are contributors—hormones, genetics, diet and lifestyle factors, including smoking, lack of exercise and tight clothing.

Massages and exercise increase blood flow so they will be of benefit in reducing cellulite, but most of all eating a balanced diet and exercising may be the best way to reduce the fat content in cells and reduce the appearance of cellulite. Of course stress should be reduced for many reasons, including keeping those hormones in check.

CHIA SEEDS

Chia is the richest plant-based source of omega 3 oils, dietary fibre, protein and antioxidants. It is available as bran, ground, seeds and oil. Your body can break down chia seeds without you having to grind them first. Once you add water to them they will go gooey, but this mucilaginous consistency is one of chia's great virtues. If you don't like this texture, then have them on their own. Just be sure to drink plenty of water afterwards, as they absorb about nine times their weight in water. If you have diverticulitis or other bowel problems, start with 10 g a day until your bowel is used to this mucilaginous fibre. If you like, you can slowly increase the amount to 30 g.

Omega 3 oils will keep the blood running smoothly, so if you're on any blood-thinning medication such as warfarin, be careful. A comparable protein to soy, chia seeds slow the conversion of carbs to sugar, making them great for weight loss and increased energy.

You don't need to take both fish oil and chia seeds. Chia seeds convert alpha-linolenic acid to EPA and DHA in the body. Fish have already done this, so when you eat fish you get the EPA and DHA.

White chia seeds have slightly more omega 3 oils than the dark ones, while the dark seeds have slightly more protein. Black seeds have more antioxidants, thereby protecting the fatty acids.

Chia seeds are naturally organic, as bugs don't really like plant oils and there's usually no need to spray them with toxic chemicals.

CHILDREN, NUTRITION

A child requires protein for growth and development, along with adequate kilojoules from good fats and oils and enough vitamins and other nutrients found in fruits, vegetables, wholegrains and sustainably caught fish. It is possible to raise a healthy vegetarian or vegan child if the parents are properly informed on how to do so. It is important that the vego/vegan child's diet is carefully considered and monitored.

Good sources of calcium, iron and protein

Calcium	Iron	Protein
Broccoli	Almonds	Chia seed
Chia seeds	Amaranth	Fruit
Chickpeas	Broccoli	Goats milk
Figs	Cherries	Grains, such as quinoa and
Parsley	Leafy green vegetables	amaranth
Sardines	Legumes such as lentils,	Legumes and pulses, such as
Sesame seeds	kidney and soybeans	chickpeas, adzuki beans
Sunflower seeds	Mulberries	and lentils
Tahini	Organic dried peaches	Nuts and seeds
Wild salmon	Organic tofu and tempeh	Organic chicken and red
Yoghurt	Pumpkins	meat
	Raisins	Soybeans and organic soy
	Raspberries	products, such as miso,
	Sea vegetables	tofu, tempeh and milk
	Sesame seeds	
	Sustainably caught fish	
	Watercress	
	Wholegrains	

Helpful foods

- protein-rich foods from non-animal sources, such as miso, legumes, tempeh and goats milk

- complex carbohydrates, such as amaranth and quinoa (both have more protein and calcium than milk) as well as wholegrains, including spelt and kamut (they are high in iron, calcium and protein), and legumes and pulses

- calcium from sesame seeds, chia seeds, chickpeas, quinoa, leafy green vegetables, fermented soy products (miso and tempeh) and broccoli

- iron-rich foods, such as organic dried peaches, sustainably caught fish, wholegrains, pumpkin, organic raisins, leafy green vegetables, sesame seeds, locally sourced sea vegetables and legumes, such as lentils, kidney and soybeans

🍲 fibre from goji berries, spelt, corn or rice crackers as well as wholegrains, legumes and fresh fruit.

Foods to avoid

🍲 junk food and excessive amounts of sweet things, especially when used as a bribe

🍲 artificial sweeteners

🍲 white sugar and its products

🍲 energy drinks

🍲 any caffeine

🍲 additives such as those starting with, but not restricted to, the letter 'e'

🍲 refined wheat and its products, as they promote allergies and mucus

🍲 raw onions and garlic, as they are too stimulating for children

🍲 too much salt, including salty spreads, as it is hard on their kidneys, increases sugar cravings and may inhibit growth

🍲 refined cooking oils and margarines, as they block fat metabolism, leading to disease later in life

🍲 too many raw foods, as they will affect the digestive system

🍲 strong spices and condiments

🍲 fruit juice, as it contains too much sugar without the fibre that whole fruit contains.

Lifestyle factors

🍲 avoid bribing children with sweets, or any food, and bargaining around food—for example, 'Eat your dinner and you can play on the computer'

🍲 encourage harmony at the dinner table

🍲 do not make more than one meal if the children don't like what you've cooked.

See also BABY, NUTRITION; KIDS' LUNCHBOXES; NUTRIENTS IN FOOD; and WATER.

CHRONIC FATIGUE
Refer to ENERGY.

CIRCULATION

Most of us, particularly women, suffer from sluggish circulation. The health of the heart is implicated here, as it is responsible for the flow of blood around your body. Therefore symptoms are high blood pressure, pins and needles or a bluish colour in the fingers and toes, or feeling cold. Smokers are highly susceptible to circulatory problems.

If you have poor circulation you are more likely to suffer from the cold during cooler months, as the cold depresses both metabolism and circulation. The cause may be due to a long-term illness, stress, the wrong diet or external factors. A lack of movement slows down your circulation, so exercise is vital. For fast results, try drinking (fresh) ginger tea. Fresh beetroot will also strengthen the heart, thereby improving circulation, while buckwheat contains a bioflavonoid called rutin, which strengthens blood vessels, thereby increasing circulation to the hands and feet.

Avoid over-eating and try to include all the different flavours in your diet—that is, sweet, salty, pungent, sour and bitter. Lemon juice, lentils, sardines and soybeans will help too. Omega 3 fatty acids will keep the blood running smoothly in cooler months—sources are sustainably caught wild salmon, sardines, anchovies and freshwater trout while vegetable sources are flaxseed oil, chia seeds, pumpkin seeds and leafy dark green veggies, such as kale, parsley and cereal grasses (wheat and barley grasses).

Too much salt slows the flow of blood and harms circulation; wind can also interrupt circulation. Pungent foods—such as legumes and seeds, oregano, rosemary, bay leaf and dill—stimulate the circulation, as do red capsicums and chestnuts. Turtle beans are the most effective here. Other foods that are known to improve circulation are pine nuts, anchovies, mussels, vinegar and black soybeans. Cherries nourish the blood and get it moving so they are great for poor circulation. Chives, lentils, mustard seeds, rhubarb, walnuts, ginger, cloves, fennel and star anise also help.

Avoid eating too many raw or cold foods and drinks; cold water should be avoided at all times. Consider also that if you are run down you may not be producing enough blood, thus decreasing circulation.

Practise a breathing technique to get the qi (energy) moving. Look into qi gong. Your breath must be going into your abdomen, not just to your chest. Avoid refined salt, animal fats (especially poor quality ones), smoking and a sedentary life.

See also AUTUMN and CARDIOVASCULAR HEALTH.

COCONUT

Isn't it great that the curtain of deceit has been lifted on coconuts? For years we were told to avoid them because of their high fat content. We now know that the fat content—the medium chain fatty acids (MFCA) that make up the coconut—helps to lower the risk of both atherosclerosis and heart disease. It is primarily the MCFA in coconut oil—the very reason we were avoiding it—that makes it so special and so beneficial.

This humble fruit—technically a drupe—provides a nutritious source of meat, water, milk and oil that has fed and nourished populations around the world for thousands of years. The coconut palm is so valued as a source of food and medicine that it has been called 'The Tree of Life'. Modern science is just catching up, discovering its healing powers.

These benefits of coconut oil can be attributed to the presence of lauric acid and its properties, such as antimicrobial, antioxidant, antifungal, antibacterial and soothing. The human body converts lauric acid into monolaurin, which is thought to help in dealing with viruses and bacteria-causing diseases, such as herpes, influenza, cytomegalovirus and even HIV.

It helps to fight harmful bacteria, such as *Listeria monocytogenes* and *Helicobacter pylori*, and also harmful protozoa, such as *Giardia lamblia*.

Avoid palm oil and sugar at all costs. It is highly refined and its cultivation destroys native habitat. Being so 'changed' makes it really bad for you. You'll find it in loads of packaged foods.

How to use it

- the oil is great for frying at high temperatures, or in almost any dish really. You can also use it to treat dandruff and as a hair pack, apply it to dry skin or add it (one tablespoon) to your bath
- coconut flour is wonderful in desserts and for coating patties
- the flesh of the young coconut is lovely when sliced finely and tossed through raw salads. Desiccated coconut, from the older coconut, is of course wonderful in bliss balls (see the recipe on page 165), truffles and all sorts of desserts, curries and vegetarian casseroles
- try coconut water in your smoothie instead of another milk; add it to vodka with a squeeze of lime juice instead of sugary, fizzy drinks; and use it to thin sauces
- coconut milk—I like it in coffee (heavenly), smoothies, curries and soups.

COLDS AND 'FLU

The common cold is caused by a viral infection that usually occurs at the change of the season or during winter. Keeping your immune system healthy by reducing stress, improving digestion and tailoring the food you eat to the season is important when trying to avoid either a cold or the 'flu. It is also important not to allow a cold to move to your chest, as this may lead to bronchitis, pneumonia or a cough that lasts for 100 days (literally).

Helpful foods

- light foods such as soup, broths and herbal teas
- honey and lemon in warm water will ease a sore throat—manuka and jelly bush honey (the Australian version) are fabulous
- garlic, shallots and onions
- garlic, cayenne pepper and shiitake mushroom broth is antiviral, antibiotic, immune-boosting and a diaphoretic (promotes sweating)
- celery and lemon juice help a cold with a fever
- foods high in bioflavonoids, such as cabbage and green capsicum
- carrots, cabbage, broccoli and parsley will soothe an aching upper back or neck
- have miso soup when the cold or 'flu starts to ease.

Foods to avoid

- heavy, fatty and oily foods
- dairy, especially if there is mucus present.

Herbal medicine

- sage tea, both gargled and drunk, will ease a sore throat
- an echinacea blend will boost your immune system—you can also take it as a preventative measure leading up to winter or when you are feeling really rundown
- St John's wort, phyllanthus or olive leaf are great antivirals
- elder for reducing phlegm
- yarrow to deal with any fever present
- astragalus is immune-enhancing and antiviral
- andrographis, a fast-acting immune booster, is great once you start feeling sick.

Spring onion, ginger and mint soup

If you catch a cold early enough, it is possible to stop it before it takes hold. Try this simple remedy for the first day of a cold.

3 shallots, white part only, roughly chopped
2 slices of fresh ginger, crushed
2 cups boiling water
small handful of fresh mint

1   Place shallots, ginger and boiling water in a saucepan on the stove. Simmer until liquid has reduced by half. Add the mint and let cool.
2   Drink when soup is cool enough. Go to bed and keep yourself warm and let the sweating begin.
3   When the sweating stops, change your clothes and rest. Nurture yourself with light, nourishing foods.

Supplements

- zinc lozenges have proven to be effective—they clear the nasal passages, boost the immune system and fight the virus; be sure to get some without sugar
- vitamin C with bioflavonoids in large doses—start on 500 milligrams every few hours (you can increase to one gram taken three to six times a day but stop if you get diarrhoea)
- propolis lozenges are useful for a sore throat
- bee pollen and royal jelly (check for allergy) have antibiotic properties so they will help ward off a cold or the 'flu; use them mindfully as they are the bees' food.

Lifestyle factors

- keep warm
- rest
- reduce overall stress in your life
- a terrible shock can significantly lower your immune system, making you more susceptible to infection, so take extra care of yourself during these times
- avoid cigarettes, alcohol and recreational drugs
- let someone look after you—no need for martyrdom when you're sick; if no one offers, consider asking for help.

Essential oils

To clear nasal passages, use a steam inhalation (boiling water in a basin with a towel over your head) with a few drops of essential oils, such as eucalyptus, peppermint, thyme, lemon, rosemary, tea tree or lavender.

See also AUTUMN, FEVER, IMMUNITY, STRESS and WINTER.

CONCEIVING NATURALLY

Infertility is described as the inability, after twelve months of intercourse, to conceive at the time of ovulation. It is often difficult to pinpoint the exact cause, as there are so many factors to consider. Stress, fear of parenthood and psychological issues along with medical causes need to be considered.

The most common causes of female infertility are failure to ovulate, blocked fallopian tubes, PCOD (see *Polycystic ovarian disease*), endometriosis, fibroids and increased age. For men, the cause can be low sperm count or motility, or an anatomical abnormality (usually a dilated vein of the spermatic cord). In some cases sexually transmitted diseases (STDs) can also be the cause.

The health of your child is determined at the time of conception, so it is important for both partners to be in peak physical condition. As it takes many months to improve your health on a deep level, it is recommended that preparation for pregnancy starts three to six months before conception.

BOTH OF YOU

Helpful foods

- everything you eat really should be organic
- essential fatty acids (EFAs), such as flaxseed, almonds, pecans, hazelnuts, sesame seeds, sunflower seeds, pumpkin seeds, walnuts, avocado, leafy green vegetables and organic soy products—your body can't provide EFAs and the food sources need to be unprocessed and unrefined
- foods high in zinc—wheatgerm, miso, pumpkin seeds, oysters, alfalfa, sardines, legumes, mushrooms, pecans, sustainably caught seafood, soybeans, sunflower seeds and wholegrains
- foods high in the B vitamins—wholegrains such as oats, brown rice and quinoa
- foods high in vitamin E, such as leafy dark green vegetables, legumes, nuts and seeds and their oils, soybeans, wheatgerm and wholegrains.

Foods to avoid

- processed, junk and fast foods
- white sugar
- gluten—the protein in wheat
- animal fats
- refined or processed oils
- irradiated foods from Europe and anything from Japan; eat locally as much as you can.

Supplements

- selenium
- vitamin E—known as the 'sex vitamin', as it carries oxygen to the sex organs and keeps hormones balanced
- zinc—important for both sperm health and the optimal functioning of reproductive organs
- B complex—important for reproductive health and the reduction of stress.

Lifestyle factors

- keep your liver well by avoiding animal fats, smoking (including passive smoking and marijuana), alcohol and too much coffee (especially instant)
- avoid excess heat from saunas, spas and vigorous exercise, as it may lead to reduced sperm count and changes in ovulation
- avoid alcohol, as it may lead to reduced sperm count in men and can prevent the implantation of the egg in women
- in case a woman has developed antibodies to her partner's sperm, use a condom for 30 days, then have intercourse at the time of ovulation
- avoid radiation by using an ear piece on your mobile phone and by not using computers or other electronic devices on your lap
- remove all chemicals from your life, both at work and at home. Cleaning, skincare and body products, room deodorisers, everything.

WOMEN

Helpful foods

- the 'Helpful foods' listed above for 'Both of you'
- vitamin B12—important for red blood cell formation and growth—is essential both for fertility and during pregnancy (the pill, smoking,

alcohol, coffee, stress or liver problems are associated with a deficiency of vitamin B12). Sources are miso paste, soy sauce, tempeh, sourdough bread, shiitake mushrooms, spirulina and chlorella

- a balanced diet high in fruit, vegetables, wholegrains, good oils and mainly plant-based protein.

Foods to avoid

- the 'Foods to avoid' listed above for 'Both of you'
- too many figs.

Herbal medicine

- damiana (adrenal tonic); ladies mantle and raspberry leaf (both these are uterine tonics); dong quai (general reproductive tonic); false unicorn root and wild yam (oestrogenic); licorice and paeonia (ovarian tonic); and motherwort (for the anxiety associated with motherhood)
- *Vitex agnus-castus* (chaste tree), which balances hormones, thereby regulating the menstrual cycle and ovulation.

Supplements

- folic acid for foetal growth and development—this is best taken with vitamin C and B12, ideally a few months before you fall pregnant.

Lifestyle

- the 'Lifestyle factors' listed above under 'Both of you'
- use 'organic' tampons, not just cotton. Ideally, use organic pads instead; don't use any bleached sanitary products.

MEN

Helpful foods

- the 'Helpful foods' listed above under 'Both of you'

◈ a balanced diet high in fruit, vegetables, wholegrains, good oils and mainly plant-based protein.

Foods to avoid

◈ the 'Foods to avoid' listed above under 'Both of you'.

Lifestyle factors

◈ the 'Lifestyle factors' listed above under 'Both of you'

◈ consider having your sperm tested for motility, health and quantity

◈ avoid vigorous exercise, hot tubs and saunas, which all reduce sperm count

◈ reduce stress

◈ recent illness or prolonged fever may reduce sperm count

◈ antidepressants may decrease sperm count

◈ avoid recreational drugs

◈ some prescription drugs can cause infertility, even impotence

◈ reduce exposure to toxins

◈ avoid excessive heat.

Herbal medicine

◈ damiana is known to increase testosterone and libido

◈ ginseng, sarsaparilla, saw palmetto and yohimbe all enhance sexual function in men

◈ astragalus has been known to stimulate sperm production

◈ tribulus is specific here for improving virility, sperm health and vitality, libido and all things relating to the male reproductive system.

Supplements

◈ the 'Supplements' listed above under 'Both of you'

◈ vitamin C to keep sperm motile.

See also Folic acid, Lactation and Pregnancy.

CORN

Corn promotes healthy teeth and gums, helps kidneys and sexual problems, and improves digestion. Corn is harder to digest than some other foods, so be sure to chew it properly or buy it as a meal—polenta or semolina—or as a puff. These gluten-free foods are cheap and nutritious.

See also WHOLEGRAINS.

CRAMPS AND SPASMS

Whether it is a random cramp that wakes you during the night, restless leg syndrome or an eye or lip twitch, the reason for the spasm is probably a magnesium deficiency. It's not surprising to find that most of us have this mineral deficiency, as magnesium is lost through stress, sweat, smoking and processed grains. Good sources of magnesium include complex carbohydrates (wholegrains, micronutrients, vegetables, nuts and seeds, beans and legumes) and locally sourced sea vegetables. Epsom salts baths are fabulous for easing cramps and spasms, as the salts are magnesium oxide. For a really relaxing bath, add some lavender leaves or oils.

Lemon juice will help too if the cramp is associated with a deficiency of fluid. Cramps and spasms may also be due to a clogged liver resulting from too much fat in your diet. Remember, you need calcium together with magnesium, so consider taking a supplement of both just to get your levels up, then be mindful of getting enough from your diet. Be sure you are drinking enough clean water, as dehydration is also a common cause. Potassium needs to be considered also.

See also LIVER, MAGNESIUM and SLEEP.

CYSTITIS

Cystitis, also referred to as a bladder infection, is an infection in the urinary tract. It is most often bacterial. As women have a shorter urethra, they tend to suffer from it more, although it does occur in men. (In men, cystitis may signal a more serious problem.) Cystitis isn't usually a serious threat, more of an annoyance. However, if left untreated it can lead to a kidney infection, which can be serious, requiring treatment with antibiotics.

The symptoms of cystitis include burning, urgency and frequency of urination, the feeling you have to empty your bladder even after urination, fever, increased thirst and cloudy urine with a strong odour. Sometimes there is blood in the urine.

Helpful foods
- echinacea, which is anti-inflammatory, to boost immunity
- garlic is a good antibiotic and immune enhancer
- parsley, celery and watermelon are natural diuretics
- include miso soup and cooling juices, such as celery and carrot and broths.

Foods to avoid
- acidic foods, such as animal meat, dairy, sugar and grains
- yeast
- caffeine, as it causes the bladder muscles to contract, resulting in painful spasms
- alcohol
- tap water—drink only pure water
- citrus fruits, as they will make your urine alkaline, helping bacteria to grow
- milk chocolate and refined or processed foods, including white flour and sugar.

Herbal medicine
- golden seal for inflammation of the mucous membranes and because it is antimicrobial

- dandelion leaf, a diuretic
- marshmallow root, which acidifies urine
- uva ursi, a urinary tract antiseptic, astringent for the lower gastro-intestinal tract and a diuretic
- buchu, a urinary antiseptic and infection fighter
- corn silk, a diuretic that soothes urinary mucosa.

Supplements

- vitamin C—one to two grams every two hours during and a few days after the infection, then slowly ween down to two to three grams per day
- acidophilus to encourage healthy gut flora
- cranberry juice, unsweetened—it contains hippuric acid, which inhibits bacterial growth and acidifies urine (if you can't get it without sugar, then get a supplement).

Lifestyle factors

- drink at least 3 litres of pure water at room temperature each day—this will increase urine flow and help rid the body of the bacteria
- maintain healthy gut bacteria by following the diet set out in *Candida*
- improve your immunity
- resolve any unresolved emotions, especially feelings of resentment and frustration (liver), fear and anxiety (kidney)
- eat lightly
- empty your bladder before and after sexual intercourse and exercise
- tampons may aggravate this condition, especially if you suffer from cystitis regularly
- avoid using soap on your genitals

- be sure to keep faecal matter away from your vagina by maintaining good hygiene and wiping from front to back after emptying your bladder or bowels
- make a broth out of barley and the silk from a fresh cob of corn, simmer and cool slightly, then drink as a tea (you can do this a couple of times a day when infection is acute and once a week for maintenance).

See also CANDIDA, IMMUNITY and WINTER.

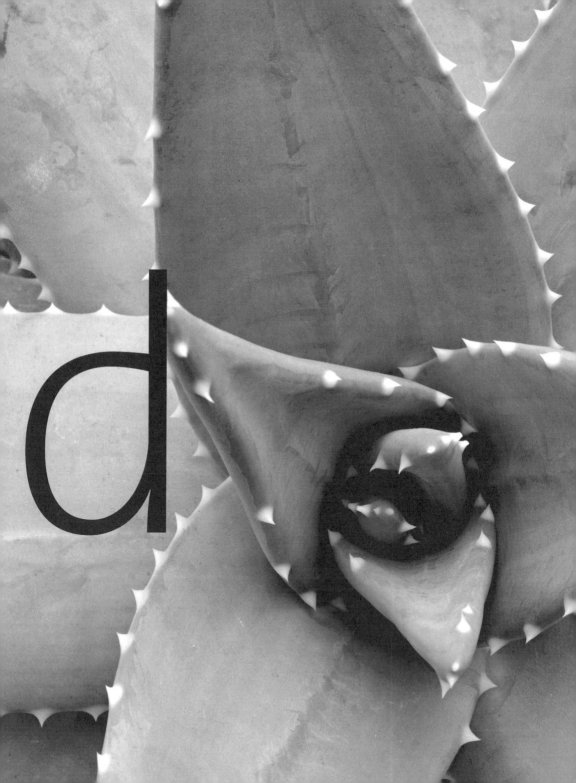

DASHI

Stock used as the base of miso. It is available from health food stores and some supermarkets. Consists of shiitake mushrooms, kombu and bonito (fish) flakes. There is a vegetarian option available.

DIABETES, TYPE 2

There are two types of diabetes—juvenile (type 1) and mature onset (type 2). Ten per cent of diabetics suffer from the former and the condition is controlled by regular injections of insulin. Type 2 diabetes, however, can be delayed or prevented through diet and lifestyle. Here I shall be discussing type 2.

Diabetes occurs because the body is unable to process sugar effectively. The pancreas produces insulin, which is attracted to cells in the body that are running short of energy. Insulin combines with glucose, then enters the cell. In diabetes type 2 the cells do not respond to the insulin, and medication in the form of tablets can make the cells respond. However, it is far preferable to prevent the onset of diabetes in the first place.

The early symptoms of diabetes include excessive tiredness, thirst, excessive passing of urine, weight loss for no apparent reason, itchy rashes, pins and needles, and blurred vision. An appropriate diet is absolutely essential for all diabetics, as glucose levels need to be kept at a constant level. Therefore, eating foods that maintain and regulate your blood sugar levels is important for prevention, as is maintaining a normal body weight.

Helpful foods

- grains and legumes, such as chickpeas, fresh corn, kamut, millet, miso, mung beans, oats, rice, soy products, spelt and wholewheat—chewed well
- seeds such as chia, sesame and flaxseed

- fruit and vegetables, such as asparagus, avocado, blueberry, carrot, grapefruit, Jerusalem artichoke, lemon, lime, pear, plum, radish, turnip and yam
- high-fibre foods such as raw cacao powder, chia seeds, psyllium husks, nuts, wholegrains, legumes and vegetables.

Foods to avoid
- natural and synthetic sweeteners, saturated fats, processed sugars, dairy, denatured foods such as genetically modified ones, salty or spicy foods and complex food combinations
- moderate your protein intake—when protein levels rise, so does the need for sugar in the body.

Herbal medicine
- gymnema, which is used extensively in India for blood sugar issues, helps to close the taste buds that detect and crave sweet foods, thus helping to balance blood sugar.

Lifestyle factors
- eat smaller, more frequent meals to help the body stimulate insulin
- chew your complex carbohydrates—these foods become sweeter the longer you chew them
- maintain your weight within the normal range
- exercise—it is of vital importance.

See also BLOOD SUGAR, BREAD, CARBOHYDRATES, ENERGY, FIBRE and WEIGHT LOSS.

DIGESTION

Most of us will complain of digestive problems at one time or another. Often all it takes is a change of diet to one of whole foods and fewer acidic foods, along with reduced stress levels and chewing properly. Some medication can also cause problems, so if this occurs check with your healthcare professional. Symptoms of digestive complaints in the upper gastrointestinal tract include indigestion, reflux, belching, peptic ulcers, hyper-acidity and halitosis (bad breath). In the lower tract you may experience nausea, constipation, diarrhoea, diverticulitis, irritable bowel syndrome, flatulence, coeliac disease, enteritis (inflammation of the intestines), colitis, bloating and lethargy.

Recommendations for better digestion

Chew Pre-digestion starts in the mouth. This is the most important factor to consider, so chew your food well. Chewing also lowers the acidic level of the food.

Avoid complex food combinations It is difficult for our bodies to digest too many food groups, so try to eat your carbohydrates and protein separately. Don't use too many flavourings, such as sauces and spices, in one meal.

Don't eat late at night After 8 p.m. your body goes into 'absorption' phase. Food and alcohol should be consumed between midday and 8 p.m. After that, only fruit, fruit juices and herbal teas should be consumed. Any food you do eat after 8 p.m. will sit in your digestive tract all night, and you will wake up feeling heavy, foggy and annoyed. I suggest you do not eat a carbohydrate- or protein-rich breakfast. I know this is controversial, but try a fruit breakfast for a month and see how you feel. Diabetics and children would do better eating a heartier breakfast, including complex carbohydrates and/or protein.

Notice how you feel before eating If you're stressed or are not hungry, then *don't* eat. Recent research has shown that high levels of cortisol (stress hormone) contribute to a 'shutting down' of digestion. Instead, eat foods that are easy to digest, such as soups and broths. Miso is fantastic, as it is loaded with nutrients and very easy to digest (it will also bring your energy back into your body if you're feeling scattered or 'high').

Eat bitter foods Stomach juices are stimulated when a message is received by a part of your brain called the hypothalamus. This message is received when the tongue detects a 'bitter' flavour (aperitifs such as lemon, lime and bitters and Campari® are used for this reason). Bitter foods include rocket, endive, alfalfa, romaine lettuce, rye, vinegar, white pepper, watercress, celery and asparagus.

Cook at home and smell the aromas Smell and sight is another way to get those stomach juices stimulated.

Eat complex carbohydrates These help with intestinal action. Examples of complex carbohydrates are fruit and vegetables, nuts and seeds, and legumes and wholegrains. Their fibre helps to keep the digestive tract functioning smoothly but they need to be chewed very well.

Avoid refined/processed foods When it comes to good digestive health, there is no place for these foods—they are very difficult to process.

Exercise Moving regularly keeps the body's organs healthy and vital.

Drink loads of clean water Drink water separately from meals, as most foods take much longer than water to move through your stomach—too many liquids with meals forces undigested food out of the stomach before it has been digested. Avoid tap water and drink no more than two to three litres per day, depending on the season.

Eat slowly Give your gut time to do its work. Those people who follow a macrobiotic diet chew each mouthful 400 times—even soup!

Help your body absorb fats Pickles assist in the absorption of fats although, due to their high salt and vinegar content, they should be eaten only in small amounts. Whenever you're eating a cooked food, eat a raw food such as pickles or sauerkraut. Daikon is also helpful for processing fats.

Cooking beans It is always better to soak any pulse overnight to remove any gas. Adding a sea vegetable called kombu to the soaking water makes pulses easier to digest. While some protein is lost in soaking, the remaining protein is about twice as digestible. When cooking beans, discard the kombu, or chop it up and put it back with the beans. If kombu is unavailable, add wakame or arame (from New Zealand or Australia, not from Japan).

Inflammatory foods Those foods that cause inflammation include animal fats (dairy and red and white meat), wheat, coffee, alcohol, warming foods such as garlic and spices, and the Nightshade family of vegetables, including capsicum, potatoes, tomatoes, eggplant and chillies. The effect of the Nightshade family is somewhat neutralised by cooking with salt or miso. Red potatoes have the mildest effect. Eating these foods will aggravate conditions such as eczema, asthma, hayfever, arthritis, sinus, irritable bowel syndrome and skin problems.

Soy products Soybeans contain a trypsin (digestive enzyme) inhibitor, which may be destroyed by long soaking and cooking. This may explain why in the Orient they are processed into readily digestible products—bean curd (tofu), soymilk and fermented products. Unfermented soy products such as milk and tofu are very difficult for our bodies to digest and should be eaten in moderation—only three to four times a week. On the other hand, fermented soy products are very easy for your digestive tract to deal with, so eating them regularly is a good idea as they are packed with essential nutrients such as protein, calcium and iron along with a good deal of B vitamins. These products include tempeh, natto miso and miso paste.

Avoid refined wheat Refined and processed wheat causes a variety of symptoms, including weight gain, indigestion, diabetes, cardiovascular complaints, constipation or diarrhoea, hayfever, sinusitis, irritable bowel syndrome, candidiasis, diabetes or hypoglycaemia. Grains such as kamut and spelt are wheat grains that are easy to digest. Millet, amaranth, quinoa and rye are highly nutritious, often higher in essential minerals, vitamins, complex carbohydrates and protein than animal products, and are easily digested, making them preferable food choices.

See also ACIDOSIS, CARBOHYDRATES, GLUTEN INTOLERANCE, IRRITABLE BOWEL SYNDROME, PULSES (LEGUMES), SOY PRODUCTS and WATER.

DRIED FRUIT AND SULFUR DIOXIDE

Unless stated otherwise, dried fruit contains a preservative called sulfur dioxide, which inhibits the growth of micro-organisms, prevents discoloration of some foods and extends the shelf life of products. It's also added to fruit juices, vinegar, processed meat and wine, just to name a few.

Sulfur dioxide has been linked to asthma, allergies and cancer. The 'Acceptable Daily Intake' for a ten-year-old weighing 21 kg is only 15 mg of sulfite per day. So how much are you and your kids consuming?

- one dried apricot—16 g
- half a thin sausage—8 mg
- one glass of cordial—5 mg
- hot chips—1 mg.

Allergies The Cleveland Clinic reports people who are allergic to sulfites could experience anaphylaxis, a serious life-threatening allergic reaction to the chemical. If you are allergic to sulfites, avoid eating dried fruits preserved with sulfur dioxide.

Asthma Also according to the Cleveland Clinic, sulfur dioxide may cause asthma symptoms, including wheezing, difficulty in breathing and life-threatening reactions. It states that most reactions are a result of inhaling sulfur dioxide generated by food containg sulfites while you are eating.

Migraines According to research by Mieczyslaw Szyszkowicz, published in the *International Journal of Occupational Medicine and Environmental*

Health in 2009, exposure to sulfur dioxide increases emergency room visits for the treatment of migraine headaches.

Cancer Research by W. J. Lee, published in *Environmental Health Perspectives* in 2002, found that exposure to sulfur dioxide increases the risk of mortality from lung cancer, leukemia and non-Hodgkin lymphoma, a type of cancer that affects the white blood cells.

If the dried fruit you buy is sulfite-free, it will proudly say so on the packet. If it is organic, it will be automatically sulfite-free.

DULSE
Refer to SEA VEGETABLES.

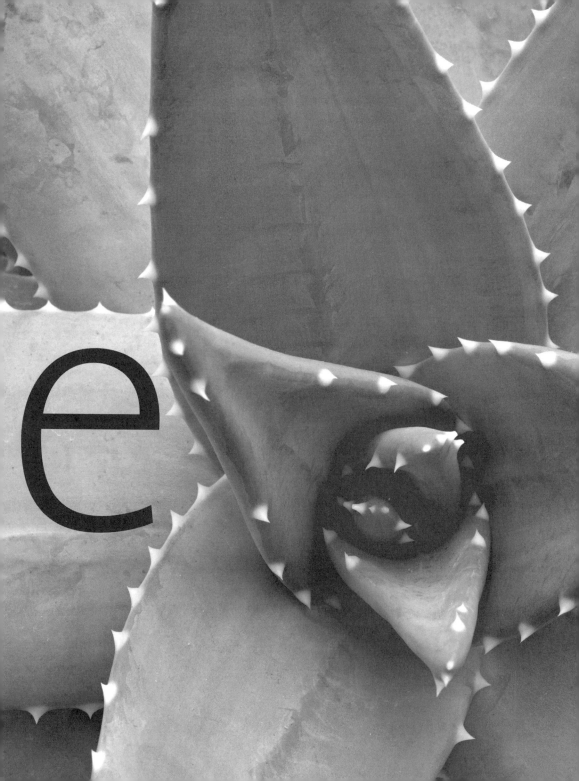

EAR PROBLEMS

Traditional Chinese medicine tells us that the kidneys govern our ears, therefore the emotions attached to them are fear and anxiety. It is interesting to note that children sometimes get earaches when school starts back after the holidays. Earaches in children are usually preceded by an allergy or respiratory infection. Wax that traps water in the canal may also be to blame.

A middle ear infection can cause perforation of the eardrum, which is not only very painful but may also result in potential hearing and bloody fluid loss. Bacteria or a virus can cause middle ear infections, and in children you should check for food allergies, as these can cause ear problems as well.

Helpful foods

- those high in betacarotene, especially carrots
- raw peanuts (organic only) are used to treat deafness (but check for allergy)
- parsley is really helpful for any ear problem
- mulberries for ringing in the ears.

Herbal medicine

- a combination of echinacea and golden seal, both gargled or taken internally, is very effective; note that golden seal is pretty hard to 'swallow', so you may need to take it as a tablet and gargle with diluted echinacea.

Supplements

- vitamin C fights infection and boosts immunity
- essential fatty acids in the diet are recommended if there is a build-up of wax—use fish oils, olive or flaxseed oils, spirulina or wheatgrass.

Lifestyle factors

- itchy ears may be a sign that parasites or candida are present
- one drop of garlic oil in the ear canal a day will usually clear an ear infection
- mullein oil, from the herb, is just as good
- chop up an onion, place it between some cloth and place over the ear
- avoid common allergens such as peanuts, wheat, dairy, corn, sugar, soy, fruit and fruit juices
- douche the nose with warm water and salt
- ear candles made with wax and herbs, available from most health food stores, are fabulous—insert one in the affected ear and the herbs will draw out the wax
- combine a few drops of tea tree oil with some warm olive oil, place a few drops into the ear canal and seal with cotton wool
- keep your immune system healthy.

See also Immunity and Winter.

ECZEMA

Eczema is not only one of the oldest known diseases but also one of the most difficult to cure. There are a variety of reasons for this, but it may be due to its relationship with the nervous system and liver. Most often, it seems blue-eyed people have a genetic predisposition to an atopic gene that causes inflammatory conditions and allergies. These are, among others, eczema, asthma, hayfever, arthritis, migraines and sinusitis. Those who suffer from any of these conditions will often tell you that when the symptoms of one disappear, another set appears.

Eczema produces symptoms such as scaling, flaking, itchiness and fluid-filled blisters that weep and ooze then form a crust. Keeping your liver functioning properly and avoiding inflammatory foods are essential for reducing symptoms. Stress is a huge trigger for eczema and other inflammatory conditions, so you need to learn how to avoid and handle stress well, and also what prompts your stress.

Helpful foods

- foods rich in omega 3 oils, such as sustainably caught deep-sea fish (cod, wild salmon, mackerel, anchovies, ocean trout and sardines), flaxseed and chia seeds and their oil, leafy dark green vegetables and organic soybean products
- unrefined sesame oil is fabulous for use both internally and externally, and sesame seeds used in salads are also of benefit—tahini is also great
- foods high in vitamin A for skin and immunity, such as carrots, kale, paw paw, sweet potato, spinach, pumpkin, leafy green vegetables and watercress
- any goats milk product is going to be very helpful, both internally and externally.

Foods to avoid

- inflammatory and acidic foods, such as red meat, dairy products, refined wheat (white bread and pasta) and the Nightshade family of vegetables (white potatoes, capsicum, eggplant, tomatoes and chillies)
- white sugar and its products
- refined fats and fried foods
- non-organic dried fruit
- processed and junk foods
- other acidic substances, such as alcohol, too much raw garlic and coffee
- too much citrus fruit.

Herbal medicine

- anti-allergens, such as baical skullcap and albizia

- immune boosters, such as echinacea (check for allergies), pau d'arco (also antifungal) and cat's claw
- chickweed applied topically (it is available as an ointment) for itchiness
- liver herbs, such as St Mary's thistle or dandelion root
- andrographis is fabulous, as it is a liver, digestive and immune-aiding herb
- schisandra, used for detoxing the liver, is great for dealing with symptoms caused by the excesses of modern living
- herbs for your nervous system are essential—try chamomile (also good for digestion), St John's wort (check with your practitioner for drug inter-reactions) and withania (also used to increase energy)
- neem, used both internally and externally, is wonderful for any skin ailment
- blood-cleansing herbs, such as yellow dock, echinacea, dandelion root and burdock (burdock has been used topically for centuries for any skin problem and internally for the liver); these herbs will also promote bowel movement
- golden seal to repair cell membranes, as an antibacterial and for its effect on the liver
- gotu kola, tea tree and calendula used topically to reduce the itch.

Supplements

- vitamin C is essential in cases of inflammation and will also help your immune system
- vitamin E may be taken internally and externally to promote healing
- blue–green micro-algae such as spirulina, wheatgrass, barley grass and chlorella
- zinc is important for the skin and the immune system.

Lifestyle factors

- be sure that your bowels move daily
- improve digestion by eating foods that are easy to digest
- avoid chemicals in cleaning and skincare products (including soap), as well as shampoos and conditioners (buy those that are sulfate-free), as these chemicals irritate the skin and liver
- keep your liver happy by eliminating the excessive amounts of toxins and preservatives found in conventionally produced fruit and vegetables, cigarettes, alcohol and processed foods
- drink purified water only and, for extra protection, buy a filter for your shower nozzle (available in health food stores)—your skin is your largest organ and it may soak up the chlorine and chemicals found in the water supply, making allergies worse
- manage stress by learning a meditation technique or by doing yoga
- exposure to the sun (as long as you avoid the hottest part of the day) and sea have been shown to be beneficial
- moderate and regular exercise is vital
- overheating will make things worse, so avoid saunas, spas, long hot showers and lots of sun
- deal with any underlying, unresolved emotional issues.

Home remedies

- to calm down the irritation, get in a tepid bath (heat makes eczema worse) with ½ cup oil (either flax or coconut). You could add a few drops of tea tree oil or lavender essential oil, or both. Rub it all over your body, focusing on where the eczema is (this is also a great remedy for dandruff); pat yourself dry
- apply raw honey (manuka is great as it is also antibacterial), umeboshi plums, a rice bran compress or fresh paw paw topically

🅿 try a bath while gently pressing a muslin cloth or laundry bag filled with oats onto your skin (oats are very soothing)

🅿 mix 1 cup goats milk powder into your bath. You could add the oils above if you like. This type of milk is anti-inflammatory and has a wonderful effect on eczema.

See also ASTHMA, FLAXSEEDS, HAYFEVER, IMMUNITY, INFLAMMATORY CONDITIONS, LIVER, OILS, SINUSITIS and STRESS.

ENDOMETRIOSIS

Once thought to affect only women over 30 years of age who hadn't had children, we now know endometriosis can occur in women of any age at any time after the onset of menstruation. It is thought to affect about 10 to 20 per cent of all women, but this estimate is likely to be higher. Women most affected may have menstrual cycles that are regularly shorter than 27 days. It also seems to be genetic—mums are likely to pass it on.

Affected women were once advised to 'have a baby' or 'a hysterectomy'. Both suggestions seemed ludicrous to me as a young girl. I was diagnosed with endometriosis at the age of 18, but I am certain I had it from the time of my first menses. (I'm sure my mother and paternal aunty had it too, but in those days they didn't have a name for it. Since I wrote the first edition of this book in 2003, my sister has also been diagnosed and told she would never conceive naturally due to her tubes being damaged by 'endo', as it is commonly called. At the age of 37 she was advised to have her fallopian tubes removed, but she ignored this advice and has since conceived naturally, giving birth to two perfect children.) I was told there was no cure but I have been symptom-free for over ten years now, and subsequent procedures have confirmed no evidence of endometriosis. I have to add that when I went off my herbs for six months or so, the symptoms started to return. Once back on my herbs for a month, they disappeared.

Endo is a condition where the cells of the endometrium (the lining of the uterus) grow in parts of the body where they shouldn't. These tissues may be found in or around the ovaries, bowel, bladder, pelvic floor, fallopian tubes and even in the nasal cavities. These misplaced tissues respond to the hormonal changes responsible for menstruation. Because they aren't where they should be—that is, in the uterus—there is no way they can be shed from the body. Instead, they are absorbed into the surrounding tissues—a painful and slow process. As each month passes, these implants grow, causing scar tissue and adhesions. This can also cause organs to stick together.

Some women with endometriosis may be symptom-free but others experience a range of symptoms, including:

- pain in the uterus, lower back and pelvis
- pain before and during menstruation
- painful intercourse
- breakthrough bleeding
- bleeding with intercourse
- intermittent pain throughout the cycle
- large clots during menstruation
- nausea, vomiting and/or constipation during menstruation
- infertility
- mood swings and/or depression
- iron deficiency due to a heavy flow.

The cause of endo is still unknown, but one thing is for sure—the pain is debilitating, as are the associated mental symptoms. Diagnosis is made through a laparoscope, usually under a general anaesthetic. Orthodox treatment involves burning off the lesions then halting menstruation by taking the contraceptive pill. This seems to be effective in some cases, for about five years at most. Treating 'endo' naturally is possible and recommended. Diet is so important here, as is exercise and stress management.

Helpful foods

- a diet free of processed oils and carbohydrates—eat wholegrains, fresh fruit and vegetables, including lots of leafy green vegetables, and raw nuts and seeds
- alfalfa contains vitamin K, which promotes normal blood clotting
- sea vegetables contain iodine, which aids in proper thyroid function
- drink only pure water—fluoridated water destroys vitamin E, which is an essential nutrient in treating endo.

Foods to avoid

- animal meat and dairy
- all saturated fats
- fried and junk foods
- additives of any kind
- refined sugar and artificial sweeteners
- alcohol, coffee and milk chocolate
- commercially produced chicken and poultry—there are too many hormones used in producing poultry so if you eat chicken, buy organic.

Herbal medicine

- dan shen for stagnant blood
- dong quai for its hormonal activity and as a general reproductive tonic—other herbs used to balance hormones are burdock, raspberry leaf and chaste tree
- dang gui is often taken alone in the East for menstrual difficulties (in the West we use *Angelica archangelica* as a substitute)
- *Vitex agnus-castus* (chaste tree) is important here, as it will regulate your cycle and balance your hormones

- *Ginkgo biloba* increases and stimulates circulation to the reproductive organs; it will also help with scar tissue
- turmeric is a good anti-inflammatory, liver tonic and oestrogenic
- calendula helps to keep lymphatics in good order, which seems to be a problem with endo
- golden seal is good for reducing inflammation in mucous membranes
- chen pi (mandarin peel) is great for improving digestion and reducing 'damp' conditions
- St John's wort is a good antidepressant and anti-inflammatory; it also helps with related sciatica
- liver herbs such as dandelion root, schisandra and St Mary's thistle are really important.

Supplements

- vitamin E aids hormonal balance and keeps blood flowing smoothly, thereby reducing stagnation and clotting; it is destroyed by tap water and the contraceptive pill
- essential fatty acids, such as evening primrose and flaxseed and fish oils from sustainably caught fish, are anti-inflammatory and help with cell rejuvenation
- iron (in liquid form for better absorption) if anaemia is present
- vitamin C, which is anti-inflammatory, for immunity and healing
- zinc for tissue repair and its immune-enhancing activity
- kelp for its mineral content and its role in thyroid function
- magnesium for the pain involved with menstruation—take it for the whole of your cycle, preferably with calcium.

Lifestyle factors

- warming your body during menstruation is important—take long baths with essential oils such as lavender, black pepper and bergamot; for period pain, a hot water bottle is your best friend

- liver stagnation is usually associated with endo, so keep your liver functioning well (see *Liver*)
- taking the contraceptive pill only 'hides' the symptoms and may cause candida, which is not easy to eliminate, so avoid taking the pill
- avoid using tampons, as they may make endo worse by preventing a good flow—Rad Pads®, although they can be impractical and messy, are great
- exercise—walking, yoga, qi gong and swimming—is really important and it *must* be regular
- if you suffer from painful menstruation, see a gynaecologist—severe period pain is not normal
- strive for emotional clarity—stress definitely makes the symptoms worse
- during menstruation, avoid physical and emotional stress
- read *The Red Tent* (1997) by Anita Diamant
- abstain from sex during menstruation—let it flow
- include dill, marjoram, black pepper and ginger in your cooking
- check for hypothyroidism
- period pain may contribute to the spread of endometrial tissue, so take steps to reduce the pain, don't endure it!
- consider not putting off having a baby if you're in a position to do so.

See also Candida, Conceiving naturally, Liver, Magnesium, Menstruation, Oestrogen, Oils, Premenstrual tension, Sea vegetables and Thyroid.

ENERGY

Many of us feel lethargic and tired at least some of the time. But for others, lethargy is part of their everyday lives. It is a big concern in our community, as conditions such as chronic fatigue syndrome and syndrome X are common diagnoses. Why do so many of us feel exhausted? And is there anything we can do about it?

There are various reasons for chronic (long-term, underlying) fatigue, but dietary considerations and lifestyle choices are leading causes. Fatigue is not an illness; it is merely a symptom of an underlying imbalance that must be addressed. These imbalances may be due to anaemia, hypoglycaemia (low blood sugar), allergies or digestive problems such as malabsorption. Of course, a high-stress lifestyle is a major contributing factor, as the stomach shuts down when you produce high levels of cortisol and adrenalin (stress hormones), which results in malabsorption of nutrients.

Deciding to buy organic will really lighten the toxic load in your body, thereby exponentially increasing your energy levels, as will removing chemicals from your home and your workplace.

Qi (pronounced chee) is your life force or energy. A person with good qi gets things done, has a clear mind and also has free-flowing blood circulating around their body. Those with good qi don't suffer from obstructions in their bodies. These obstructions can manifest as tumours, cysts, obesity, clots and a variety of other symptoms, including viruses. Your diet has a lot to do with how well your qi is circulating, as do your stress levels. Sources of qi include your food and the air you breathe (good kidney health is probably the most important factor). Your attitude towards life will determine how well you utilise your qi.

Helpful foods

- to increase energy (qi)—mussels, oysters, prawns, herring, sardines and mackerel
- wholegrains, such as rye, barley, spelt, millet, amaranth, brown rice, quinoa and oats
- sunflower seeds, sweet potato, watercress and squash
- lots of sustainably caught fish instead of meat and chicken
- fruit, vegetables and grains
- eat a small amount of raw food daily—juices are good for this

⍻ shiitake mushrooms (high in vitamin B12) to help with anaemia and fatigue.

Foods to avoid
⍻ refined carbohydrates, such as white flour, bread and pasta
⍻ refined sugar and its products, and artificial sweeteners
⍻ animal fats, including meat and dairy
⍻ refined vegetable oils and margarines.

Herbal medicine
⍻ Siberian ginseng—not to be taken if you are already hyped up, over-stimulated, have any heart problems or are hypoglycaemic
⍻ withania, especially for depletion and anaemia
⍻ licorice—not to be taken by those with high blood pressure
⍻ rhodiola is a great adrenal herb for physical and emotional stress
⍻ gotu kola is an age-old remedy for adrenal rejuvenation, and has other virtues
⍻ damiana is an antidepressant that also helps with libido
⍻ *Ginkgo biloba*, as a circulatory stimulant
⍻ liver herbs, such as St Mary's thistle, dandelion root and schisandra.

Supplements
⍻ royal jelly and bee pollen—be careful with these, as some people are allergic to them, especially asthmatics
⍻ coenzyme Q10 to help put oxygen into your cells
⍻ a vitamin A and B complex injection may be necessary in severe cases (check with your GP).

Lifestyle factors
⍻ drink pure water
⍻ avoid caffeine, alcohol and guarana

- especially avoid so-called 'energy drinks'
- exercise in moderation and regularly
- address emotional stress
- check the fatigue doesn't stem from boredom or depression
- avoid drugs and tobacco
- don't eat after 8 p.m.
- check for food intolerance—the likely offenders will be wheat and/or dairy
- check your thyroid health
- check for allergies
- get adequate rest
- enjoy your life
- don't work all the time
- keep your liver in good order
- consider having your blood tested—it's a good idea to know what's going on in your body so anything sinister can be eliminated.

See also DIGESTION, LIVER, OILS, SLEEP and WEIGHT LOSS.

EYES

Eye problems? Think vitamin A and consider the health of your liver, and of your immune system of course. Traditional Chinese medicine tells us that the liver controls the eyes and the tendons, so liver health is vital for good eye health.

Helpful foods

- organic soybeans promote clear vision
- celery is good for eye inflammations
- cucumber slices laid directly onto the eyelids help tired, hot, inflamed, swollen, dry or irritated eyes
- black sesame seeds help blurred vision; also try black tahini

- broccoli, cabbage and cauliflower are necessary for liver health
- leafy green vegetables, squash, watercress and sunflower seeds are also good
- carrot juice is full of vitamin A.

Foods to avoid
- excess salt—use only sea salt
- refined sugar or flour.

Herbal medicine
- for tired, sandy, itchy, inflamed or sore eyes, use calendula, chamomile, eyebright or golden seal as an eyewash—this is also great for conjunctivitis
- echinacea and eyebright taken internally will help any eye problem
- bilberry is good for poor vision and eyestrain
- shepherd's purse brightens the eyes and benefits the liver
- a raspberry leaf tea compress will relieve redness and irritation
- green or chamomile tea bags soothe tired eyes.

Supplements
- dry eyes need essential fatty acids such as spirulina and flaxseed oil, as well as vitamins A and C, and antioxidants such as selenium and grape seed extract
- B vitamins are needed for eyes and also the metabolism
- potassium controls fluid, so take it if you have puffy eyes
- vitamin A is of the utmost importance for maintaining proper intra-ocular fluid
- vitamin E is for healing and immunity
- low zinc levels have been linked to retinal detachment and vision loss
- conjunctivitis requires zinc and vitamins B, A and C

- itchy eyes may be due to allergies or a deficiency in either vitamin B or essential fatty acid
- spots in the visual field are usually related to liver insufficiencies.

Lifestyle factors

- exercise regularly
- adrenal exhaustion can sometimes show up as black circles under the eyes
- avoid eyestrain and exercise your eyes by looking as far into the distance as you can for 15 seconds several times a day
- avoid smoking and excessive alcohol consumption
- get adequate sleep
- it is important to avoid spreading an infection, so use separate eye baths for each eye and sterilise all implements before use
- use natural skincare products around your eyes
- avoid using harsh chemicals around your eyes—if you are having eye problems, eyelash tinting or eyelid tattooing may need to be re-evaluated.

See also IMMUNITY, INFLAMMATORY CONDITIONS, LIVER, ORGANS AND ASSOCIATED EMOTIONS and SOY PRODUCTS.

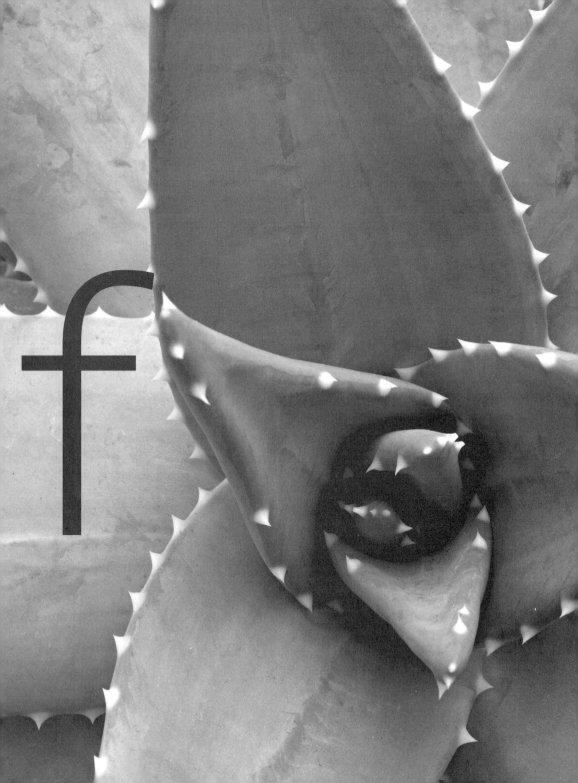

FERTILITY

Refer to CONCEIVING NATURALLY.

FEVER

A fever occurs when your body is invaded by nasty microbes. Your immune system, which is on constant alert for this kind of invasion, will sense an intrusion and release proteins. This reaction tells your brain to turn up the heat to rid your body of the microbes, mainly through the skin.

Having a fever in some cases is dangerous, as it may be too strong or last too long, affecting the brain and dehydrating the body. If the fever is suppressed, the disease will move deeper, and possibly become chronic (long-term). A mild fever of, say, about 38–39°C doesn't need to be controlled, rather it should be left to do its job. A temperature of 37°C is considered safe, but one of 39°C starts to become dangerous. This situation tends to inspire fear and sometimes panic, especially in parents of young children.

Many parents rely upon ear thermometers. Although they are expensive and not always accurate, they are good for tracking the fever—that is, monitoring if it is going up or down.

Helpful foods

- the diet must be light, consisting of only juices and teas—if you're hungry, eat only fruit, vegetables and miso
- diaphoretic herbs such as fresh ginger, elder or yarrow are indicated here—try sipping it as a tea while you have a hot bath, then popping under your blankets (change the sheets if they become damp)
- folklore suggests a tea made out of elder, yarrow, peppermint and a pinch of cayenne, which can be sipped, or added to your bath, or used as a foot bath
- a valuable folk remedy is to add lemon and/or rosehips (vitamin C) and honey to tea

- grapefruit (and, to a lesser degree, orange) pulp and juice brewed as a tea—that is, simmered for ten minutes—can be sipped slowly to help a mild fever; also try mung beans or green tea
- soybeans and alfalfa have been traditionally used to reduce fever
- kudzu combined with rice syrup or apple juice is useful. This is made by dissolving the kudzu in a little hot water, then adding the syrup or juice and letting it cool.

Supplements

- vitamin C is an effective treatment, as it flushes out toxins and reduces fever
- royal jelly is good too, unless you are allergic to it.

Essential oils

- black pepper, lavender and peppermint are helpful, either added to your bath or mixed with oil and rubbed directly onto your body.

See also AUTUMN, COLDS AND 'FLU, HEADACHES, IMMUNITY and WINTER.

FIBRE

Fibre is a very important form of carbohydrate. It isn't absorbed by digestive enzymes, so most of it moves through the gut and ends up in the stool. It holds onto water, helping to form softer stools, thereby preventing constipation, thus haemorrhoids. By including enough fibre in your diet, you are reducing your risk of colon cancer. This may be due to having a cleaner colon because you are eliminating more thoroughly. Fibre also lowers cholesterol, decreasing your risk of heart disease. In addition, it also helps to keep your blood sugar stable and assists with weight loss. The fact that it removes toxic metals from your body through the bowel is a bonus.

The bulk of your diet should come from complex carbohydrates. As the processing and refining of food removes most of its natural fibre, it's little wonder we see increasing numbers of people suffering from diabetes and digestive, weight and heart problems. Good sources of fibre are wholegrains such as brown rice and quinoa, agar agar, nuts and seeds, prunes, rice bran, fresh fruit and vegetables, flaxseeds (these are especially good), legumes, oatmeal and sesame seeds. Psyllium seeds are a great intestinal cleanser.

If you take supplemental fibre, be sure that you take it separately from other supplements and medications, as it may lessen their effect. It is important to drink one to two glasses of water after you take the supplement, otherwise it will harden like a rock in your digestive tract, causing constipation and pain.

There are popular fibre supplements you can buy in supermarkets and pharmacies, but always read the label on these. They are either artificially sweetened and coloured or contain added sugar. They are expensive and usually not presented in recycled packaging.

Good sources of fibre are wholegrains such as brown rice, millet, amaranth and oats; seeds such as quinoa; agar agar; raw cacao; maca powder; goji berries; prunes; rice bran; fresh fruit and vegetables; flaxseed and chia seeds (especially good); legumes; slippery elm; LSA; and sesame seeds. Psyllium seeds are a great intestinal cleanser.

See also BLOOD SUGAR; CANCER; CARBOHYDRATES; CARDIOVASCULAR HEALTH; DIABETES, TYPE 2; DIGESTION; HAEMORRHOIDS; and WATER.

FLAXSEEDS

Also known as linseeds, flaxseeds have become increasingly popular over the past twenty years, and with good reason. They contain ALA oils that turn into omega 3 oils in your gut. They are the richest source of omega 3 fatty acids and they also contain a good deal of magnesium, potassium, fibre, B vitamins, protein and zinc. Flaxseeds strengthen immunity, keep the arteries and heart clean, reduce the pain and swelling so often associated with arthritis, and lower blood cholesterol. They are very useful in weight loss, for cell renewal, depression (including post-natal), migraine, hives and other allergies, enlarged prostate, liver function, phlegm reduction, stomach ulcers, period pain, hormone balance, irritable bowel syndrome, PMT, ADHD and HIV/AIDS.

LSA—a mixture of ground-up linseeds, sunflower seeds and almonds—is popular with menopausal women around the world due to its oestrogenic effect and essential fatty acid content. The problem with buying LSA is that it goes rancid quite quickly after grinding. I know it's inconvenient, but if you can buy the three ingredients separately and whiz them in a coffee or spice grinder as you need them, you will get the most out of your purchase. When choosing flaxseed oil, make sure it hasn't been exposed to heat, light or air, as this will cause oxidation. Buy one in a dark bottle. Once opened, it will be at its best before two weeks but starting to deteriorate after this. Try to use it all within six weeks of opening the bottle. If yours is past this use-by-date, don't throw it away—use it as a scalp massage for a flaky scalp, or put it in the bath to soften and moisturise your skin in the cooler months and to reduce the itchiness associated with eczema.

The dosage is one to three tablespoons of oil a day, which you can use instead of olive oil on your food—but please don't heat it. Or grind up the flaxseeds yourself. Add them to your breakfast, smoothies, dessert, bliss balls (see the recipe on page 165) and yoghurt.

See also Arthritis, Attention Deficit Hyperactivity Disorder (ADHD), Headaches, Irritable bowel syndrome, Oils and Premenstrual tension.

'FLU
Refer to Autumn, Colds and 'flu and Immunity.

FOLIC ACID
The B vitamin known as folic acid is very important during pregnancy, as it is required by the foetus for red blood cell formation and neural tube

growth. It also strengthens immunity by aiding white blood cell formation for both mother and child, and works best when combined with vitamins B12 and C. It is helpful in depression and anxiety. A sore red tongue is a common sign of deficiency. Good sources of folic acid are fresh fruit and vegetables. Microwaving your food will destroy it, and digestive trouble may prevent you from having adequate levels.

See also CONCEIVING NATURALLY, LACTATION and PREGNANCY.

FROZEN SHOULDER

This is a very painful and debilitating condition. Orthodox treatment recommends surgery to remove the offending nerve. The problem is, of course, this treatment isn't dealing with the underlying problem; it merely removes the symptom. The frozen shoulder is still a problem, as another nerve(s) will become affected.

It is quite a curious condition and there are many treatments and explanations given for it, unfortunately with little relief. I have noticed, however, that when you reduce acid in the body, many conditions, including this one, are reduced. Umeboshi plums are extremely helpful here, as they are highly alkaline. Eat one, or one teaspoon of the vinegar, a day. Acidic-forming foods need to be reduced and replaced with alkaline-forming foods. Chew. Drink alkaline water. Alcohol is highly acidic so it makes it worse. Bromelain, an enzyme found in pineapples and available as a supplement, is a popular treatment, as is vitamin C.

Frozen shoulder is often misdiagnosed. Be sure your spine is in alignment, as often a back issue may come out in your shoulder. And weak tummy muscles can start to affect your back. Check also for arthritis. Vitamin C and echinacea are both good anti-inflammatories.

See also ACIDOSIS and UMEBOSHI PRODUCTS.

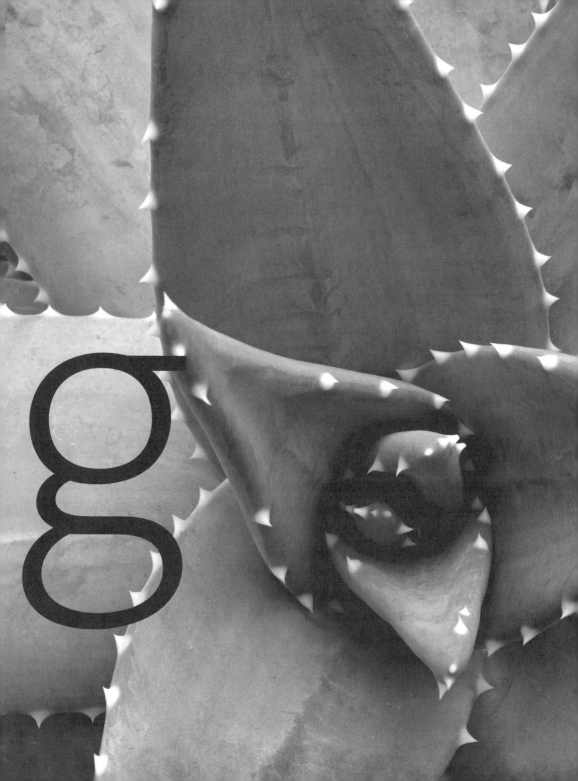

GLANDULAR FEVER

Most of us have either had glandular fever, or know someone who has had it, because it is highly contagious, airborne and transmitted through close contact such as kissing, sexual contact, or sharing cutlery or a drink bottle. This means that if you're rundown or otherwise immuno-suppressed and someone with glandular fever sneezes on you or shares your drink or food, there's a pretty good chance you will contract the virus. This is why it is so important to keep your immune system as healthy as possible.

The virus that causes this infectious disease is either Epstein-Barr (EBV) or cytomegalovirus (CMV). It can enter your cells and lie dormant until the immune system is compromised to the point where it cannot fight it. So a cold, 'flu, other virus or increased stress—physical, emotional, mental or spiritual—can often be seen as the start of the symptoms.

This virus is seen mostly in children and teenagers, but it's not exclusive to them. Incubation is about two weeks in children and one to two months in adults. This is a determined virus whose symptoms can persist for months to years. The symptoms include depression, poor concentration, anxiety, irritability, memory loss, fatigue, lethargy, general aches, joint pains, headaches, sore throat, swollen glands, fever, digestive complaints, allergies, chemical sensitivities, weight changes and respiratory complaints. A blood test is required to confirm the diagnosis. Sometimes we find out we've had glandular fever but didn't know it at the time.

Helpful foods

- shiitake mushrooms are immune-boosting and antiviral—they also help oxygen reach your fatigued cells
- barley will help oxygenate your cells
- get as much chlorophyll as you can from leafy dark green vegetables—chlorella, wheatgrass, spirulina, barley grass, rocket, kale, parsley, baby spinach, Asian greens and silver beet

🌿 foods high in fatty acids are antiviral and prevent the virus from replicating—these are leafy green vegetables, spirulina, wholegrains, sprouts, flaxseed and fish oils, and soy products.

Foods to avoid

Foods that depress the immune system—including processed and refined foods, sugar, coffee and tea, and fried and fast foods—need to be avoided and, preferably, eliminated.

Herbal medicine

🌿 immune-boosting herbs such as echinacea (which also cleans the blood), astragalus (helps with nutrient absorption) and pau d'arco (antifungal) are useful

🌿 antivirals, including olive leaf, phyllanthus and St John's wort, which is specific for glandular fever as it is effective against retroviruses; it is also an antidepressant and anti-inflammatory

🌿 liver herbs—St Mary's thistle, dandelion root, licorice (also aids digestion, lungs and eases a sore throat) or schisandra

🌿 for energy try Siberian ginseng to counteract the effects of too much stress on your body, both physical and mental, but avoid it if you have high blood pressure or hypoglycaemia or suffer from anxiety; it will also help with cellular oxygenation

🌿 digestive herbs—golden seal (also fights infection), gentian, chamomile, meadowsweet, andrographis (also for the liver and immunity) and peppermint (also improves liver function).

Supplements

🌿 chlorella has the highest amount of chlorophyll of any food and chlorophyll is immune-boosting, antifungal, antiviral and also helps oxygenation

- vitamin C is immune-boosting and fights the virus
- B vitamins are good for energy, digestion, brain function and the nervous system—consider getting an injection from your GP
- garlic acts as a natural antibiotic and immune booster, and increases oxygenation
- acidophilus is important for keeping your gut healthy
- coenzyme Q10 helps get oxygen into your cells, thereby increasing energy.

Lifestyle factors

- exercise moderately and regularly to help oxygen reach your cells, which is of vital importance—oxygen purifies and eliminates waste, yeast and parasites
- if you're too exhausted to even contemplate exercise, check out qi gong
- yoga is wonderful, as it encourages deep breathing, which also helps with oxygenation
- eat simply, avoiding complex food combinations
- don't eat until you are full—a good rule is to stop when you are two-thirds full
- try to remain positive and know that you will enjoy good health again
- rest, especially during the acute phase
- avoid antibiotics, as they are of no use unless they are needed for a secondary infection
- both the viruses that cause this condition will remain in your body for life (so they say . . .), therefore it is important to always take extra care of yourself
- there is an increased risk of gut problems, so aloe vera gel is a good idea for keeping your colon happy
- avoid sharing utensils, food, linen etc. with others and practise good hygiene—wash your hands regularly

- your liver is likely to make you very sensitive to petrol fumes, chemicals, perfumes and certain foods, so try to use natural skincare and cleaning products
- avoid habits that compromise your immunity, such as smoking, too much alcohol, recreational drugs, promiscuous sex, hating your job, negative thought patterns and a poor diet
- drink eight to ten glasses of purified water a day.

See also COLDS AND 'FLU, IMMUNITY and STRESS.

GLUTEN INTOLERANCE

Gluten is the protein in some grains that most of us have trouble digesting. If you react to gluten, avoid wheat, oats, barley and rye. Include millet, quinoa, brown rice, buckwheat and amaranth. Spelt and kamut contain gluten, but are usually easy to digest as they have not been adulterated—check with a small amount first. Avoid them if you are coeliac.

Seriously, I'm so intolerant of food manufacturers who have jumped on the marketing opportunity that is 'gluten-free'. You can buy gluten-free chicken now. What? And the products available are so highly processed and usually include so many additives that the ingredients list can barely fit on the polystyrene container. Those additives are going to do you a damn sight more harm than the appropriate amount of gluten in barley or spelt.

It's not the gluten in whole 'unchanged' grains such as spelt and kamut that's the problem. It's the modification of the wheat grain so that it now contains three to four times the amount of gluten than it used to. It's too much gluten all at once. And it's not just our bread that's been affected, but so much of what we eat—canned foods, sauces, dips and spreads, condiments, frozen meals, vacuum-sealed foods, breakfast cereals, cornflour, baking powder, crackers, biscuits, pizza, pasta, wraps, ice cream etc.

The best thing to do is cut out all types of mass-produced bread—brown, white, multigrain, soy and linseed, the works. Also remove anything from your diet that uses white or wholemeal flour to make it. You don't need to go crazy and remove *everything* with gluten but it's probably a good idea for a while, just to rid your body of gluten build-up; besides, it'll mean you're getting rid of lots processed and refined foods. Once you start to reintroduce good sources of gluten, the processed food can remain out.

Yes, you will eat a pizza again and it will contain gluten, but this will be after you've removed all gluten for a couple of weeks. Try a little bit in something like spelt sourdough bread. See if it affects you, and don't eat gluten every day. It's a good way to expand your diet and include other grains. Replace things like the white flour in your pantry with brown rice flour, which I use for thickening or coating things such as veggie patties. I use 100 per cent buckwheat noodles instead of pasta; corn or rice thins instead of wheat crackers; and pure organic ingredients for all my sauces and oils etc. That way I know I'm not consuming secret doses of modern-day wheat and gluten.

See your intolerance as a blessing rather than an inconvenience. Instead of feeling deprived of a burger, feel empowered by knowing what to eat instead.

By the way, if you've been diagnosed with coeliac disease, you are allergic to rather than intolerant of gluten. You will need to avoid gluten for the rest of your life. (The percentage of people diagnosed with coeliac disease has dramatically risen in the past few years.) In the words of John Harrison and his best-selling book—*Love Your Disease: It's Keeping You Healthy.*

See also Bread and Carbohydrates.

GOJI BERRIES

Native to the Himalayas, goji berries are the red fruits of plants in the *Lycium* genus, which are related to potatoes, tomatoes and tobacco, other plants in the Nightshade family. In English they are also known as wolfberries. Available as a dried fruit, powder or juice, goji berries have been used in traditional Chinese medicine for hundreds of years, and are now gaining popularity as a 'superfruit' because they contain so many nutrients and antioxidants. These red berries, which resemble small peppers, have been used for more than 5000 years in East Asia.

Goji berries are very high in fibre and vitamin A—they contain more betacarotene than any other food, even carrots—and, to a lesser extent, vitamin C (more than oranges per weight), calcium and iron. Goji berries are also very high in antioxidants, so they are a great anti-inflammatory and detoxer. In traditional Chinese medicine, goji is used as an immune tonic and a blood tonic. Research on their medicinal properties is being carried out around the globe.

Gojis berries don't taste great, so it's a good idea to soften them in water before adding them to smoothies, syrups or cakes. Dried goji berries are usually cooked before you eat them, so you can add them to stuffings, soups, teas, casseroles or congee. You can use them with chrysanthemum leaves as a tea.

Be sure to buy organic or at least sulfur-free goji berries, as the berries of Chinese origin have been found to have unacceptable levels of pesticides, leading to the confiscation of these products.

See also DRIED FRUIT AND SULFUR DIOXIDE.

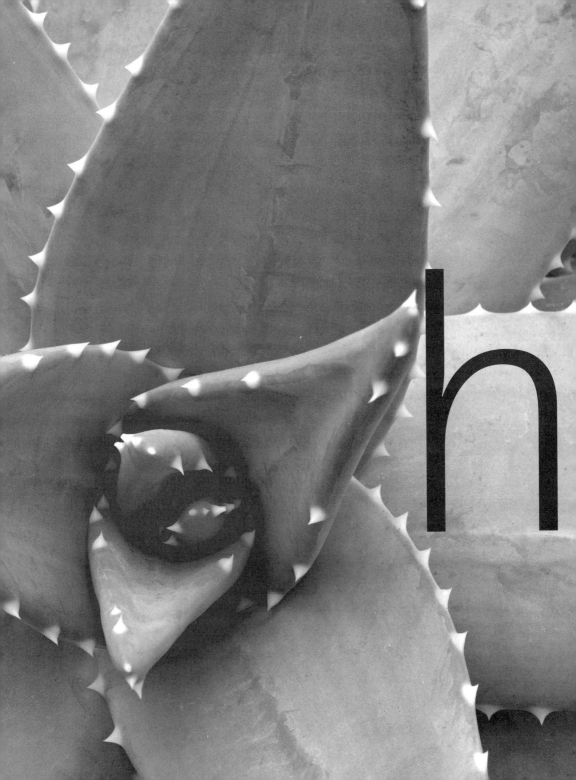

HAEMORRHOIDS

Between 50 and 75 per cent of the population have haemorrhoids, and some don't even know it. As haemorrhoids are unique to humans, a poor diet low in nutrients and fibre seems to be a contributing factor, yet again. (Being bipedal probably has something to do with it also.) Commonly known as 'piles', this condition occurs when the veins around the rectum (the lowest part of the colon) swell, causing a protrusion of veins from the anus. Similar to varicose veins, elasticity is reduced, causing the grape-like protrusions. Age is usually a predisposition, as is pregnancy, standing or sitting for too long, constipation, muscle weakness, veinous insufficiency and incorrectly performed heavy lifting. A weakness in the abdominal muscles seems to be associated also. Haemorrhoids appear to be hereditary.

There are a few different types of haemorrhoids:

- internal—usually pain-free, but can bleed; the blood is bright red in colour
- external—can be painful as they develop at the opening of the anus
- prolapsed, the result of internal haemorrhoids that have collapsed and then protruded outside—very, very painful as they discharge mucus and bleed.

The symptoms include burning, itching, pain, inflammation, swelling, irritation, discharge and bleeding.

Helpful foods

- if bleeding, include foods high in vitamin K—alfalfa and leafy dark green vegetables; eggplant has also been shown to help
- fibre-rich foods—especially apples, beetroot, cabbage, brussels sprouts, broccoli, figs, lettuce, pears, raw cacao, powder, chia seeds and goji berries—to reduce constipation and improve digestion

℞ under-ripe organic bananas are very astringent—steam the whole banana and eat it skin and all twice a day on an empty stomach—and will also help with bleeding haemorrhoids.

Foods to avoid

℞ saturated fats (mostly from animal products and junk food), as they are hard on your digestion, especially the lower colon.

Herbal medicine

℞ bupleurum (a Chinese herb) is used for prolapse of any kind

℞ grape seed extract as an antioxidant and for venous circulation

℞ horse chestnut for veinous circulation also

℞ witch-hazel is astringent—apply topically.

Supplements

℞ fibre such as psyllium husks or oat bran—be sure to drink at least one to two glasses of water straight after taking them

℞ vitamin C with bioflavonoids for healing and circulation

℞ vitamin E for proper blood clotting, circulation and wound healing

℞ vitamin B to reduce stress and digestive complaints

℞ acidophilus for good digestive health

℞ flaxseed oil to soften stools

℞ wheatgrass for liver health, gastrointestinal inflammation and poor digestion.

Lifestyle factors

℞ drink lots of purified water

℞ keep your colon clean by eliminating daily—this will relieve the pressure on the rectum

℞ don't strain when moving your bowels

- be mindful of activating your core
- warm water reduces swelling—either take regular baths or apply water topically
- exercise regularly and moderately
- avoid laxatives, as your body will start to rely on them
- learn how to lift correctly—don't hold your breath; instead exhale upon lifting.

See also CARBOHYDRATES, LACTATION, OILS and PREGNANCY.

HAIR

The health of your hair, like that of your skin and nails, comes mostly from what's going on inside you. That is to say, if your body is deprived of essential nutrients, your hair will suffer. If you use commercial shampoos and conditioners, you are doing your hair and the environment a great disservice. These products are very similar to commercial household cleaning products, so they are harsh and strip your hair and scalp of its natural oils and vitality. Go for products that are sulfate-free—there are many available.

The condition of your hair reflects the health of your kidneys. Your hair will change naturally every seven years. Hormonal changes, such as pregnancy and menopause, are also likely to affect your hair.

Helpful foods
- essential fatty acids—from wholegrains, legumes, fresh nuts and seeds, leafy dark green vegetables, spirulina, flaxseed oil and pumpkin and chia seeds—help with dry and brittle hair, improving the texture
- foods high in B vitamins for hair health and growth
- those high in vitamin C for improved circulation to the scalp
- foods high in vitamin E increase oxygen uptake and improve circulation, thereby improving hair health and growth

- zinc stimulates hair growth by improving immunity
- kelp is packed with minerals to promote growth
- protein-rich foods are important for growth
- biotin deficiency has been linked to hair loss and skin problems—foods high in biotin are brown rice, cracked wheat, peas, lentils, oats, soybeans, sunflower seeds and walnuts
- arame, hijiki and wakame promote gloss and prevent loss
- mulberries strengthen the liver and kidneys, thereby preventing premature greying and hair loss.

Foods to avoid

- raw eggs contain a protein called avidin, which binds to biotin and stops it from being absorbed—cooked eggs are okay
- sugar is highly acidic, destroying B vitamins and decreasing minerals, leading to unhealthy hair.

Herbal medicine

- apple cider vinegar together with sage as a tea, massaged into your scalp, will help hair grow
- licorice may prevent loss; avoid in cases of high blood pressure
- horsetail contains silica, which makes hair strong and shiny
- stinging nettle made into a tea and massaged into the scalp will stimulate hair follicles.

Supplements

- coenzyme Q10 improves oxygenation and circulation to the scalp.

Lifestyle factors

- use natural haircare products—commercial products will slowly but surely weaken your hair and rid it of its natural oils
- hypothyroidism can cause hair loss, so check you don't suffer from this

- stress, poor nutrition, sleep deprivation and illness will affect how your hair looks and feels
- get a good brush with soft, round bristles
- if you colour your hair, use a natural dye—available from health food stores and some salons
- be gentle with your hair when it's wet, as it will be more elastic and will break easily
- use a wide-tooth comb or brush, as fine teeth may pull out your hair
- if you are losing a lot of hair, see your healthcare practitioner
- massage your scalp regularly
- headstands, and other inverted yoga poses, encourage improved circulation to the head
- wash your hair as irregularly as you can manage, but brush it daily.

Home remedies

- for damaged hair, make a paste out of 1 egg yolk, 1 tablespoon olive oil and 1 tablespoon milk powder, massage into your scalp, leave on for 30 minutes, then rinse and wash
- for bleached or dull hair, mix together an egg and olive oil, massage into your hair, leave for 10 to 20 minutes, then wash
- to reduce dandruff, mix together olive, coconut and castor (or flax) oils with a bit of yoghurt, massage into your scalp and wrap in a hot towel for an hour—keep reheating the towel when it cools down.

See also NUTRIENTS IN FOOD and SEA VEGETABLES.

HANGOVER

The symptoms of a hangover are caused by too many toxins being forced through the liver. They are also due to the sugar content in alcohol, which sends your blood sugar way up—creating feelings of happiness and elation while under the influence—then crashing way down low the day after. This see-saw action has the same effect as eating refined sugar or carbohydrates, as the day after you will often crave more alcohol or salty, fatty foods to counteract the crash. Sugar is an 'ascending' substance energetically, which makes you feel dizzy, confused and anxious. The salt and fat you crave are 'descending'. You may be trying to 'balance' yourself by giving in to the craving, but this isn't the way to do it. These foods put extra stress on your liver and simply continue the see-saw effect.

Before the party shoes are slipped on

- have something substantial to eat
- take some dandelion root or St Mary's thistle, as this will help your liver process alcohol more efficiently.

During the party

- have a glass of water in between each drink
- try not to drink quickly, and monitor your intake
- stick to one type of drink—mixing white with red wine or spirits with beer is a recipe for a shocking day-after
- avoid pre-mixed drinks as they have a very high alcohol and sugar content.

Before bed

- your hangover will be worse if you go to bed drunk—stay up for a while
- have two to three glasses of water and leave a big glass beside your bed to drink during the night or first thing upon waking
- take some herbal medicine for the liver such as St Mary's thistle, dandelion, burdock or schisandra.

The day after

- for sugar or alcohol cravings, try one teaspoon honey
- grapefruit juice is very effective

- soak one umeboshi plum in boiling water for five minutes, drink the liquid, then eat the plum (umeboshi plums are available from health food stores)
- miso soup will balance your blood sugar and help rid your body of toxins from cigarettes
- sip on a tea of burdock, schisandra, valerian and echinacea—buy the dried herbs from a health food store
- try peppermint or ginger tea if you are experiencing nausea—umeboshi plums are also effective here
- boil orange peel from a whole orange for 30 minutes, cool, then drink the liquid
- the Romans thought wearing a celery wreath around your head could ease a hangover—perhaps because it is a cooling food and too much alcohol makes you hot
- vitamin B5 aids alcohol detox
- dandelion and St Mary's thistle help to repair damage to the liver
- the herb valerian has a calming effect on the nervous system due to its high levels of magnesium, which is often deficient in alcohol toxicity
- avoid saturated fat, fried foods and sugar
- if you're feeling agitated, sprinkle some shallots over your meal.

HAYFEVER
Refer to INFLAMMATORY CONDITIONS.

HEADACHES
Most of us will experience a headache at some time. There are many causes and various types. It is important to take into account your body type, environment, diet, hormones, stress levels and the season. When headaches are an issue, usually the health of your liver needs to be addressed. When there is too much 'heat' in the body, symptoms such as a headache will result.

Heat accumulates in your body when you consume too many fatty foods—such as animal products, processed and refined oils from junk foods and sugars—or you regularly experience feelings of anger, resentment or frustration. Therefore you need to counteract heat with cooling foods and oils. Overloading your body with toxins such as nicotine, alcohol, coffee and environmental pollutants will also make your liver heat rise, thereby giving you a headache. Common causes of headaches are:

alcohol
allergies
anxiety
chemicals
constipation
dehydration
eye problems
eye strain
fever
high blood pressure
hormonal imbalance
low blood sugar

muscle tension in the neck and back
   (often caused by sitting at a computer)
nutritional deficiencies
perfume
pollution
premenstrual tension or menstruation
   stress
sinusitis
spinal problems
teeth grinding
tension
tiredness or when detoxing
tobacco

Common triggers are:

anxiety or feelings of anger
dairy foods
dehydration
milk chocolate
MSG (monosodium glutamate)
nuts

preservatives in food
refined wheat
resentfulness or frustration
sugar
tobacco or alcohol

Types of headaches

- rear of head, usually caused by withdrawal of toxic substances, with pain that is dull, non-throbbing and worse in the cold
- frontal—caused by too much sugar, cheese, wine or prescription drugs, and dehydration or low blood sugar, with pain that is throbbing, sharp, stabbing or explosive, made worse by warmth

- side, triggered by too many oily, fatty or greasy foods, with pain that may be dull or sharp
- deep inside, usually triggered by consuming too many animal products—this is a pressure type of pain deep inside the brain.

Helpful foods

- omega 3 oils from sustainably caught fish, walnuts, locally sourced sea vegetables, chia seeds or flaxseed
- persimmon for a headache caused by a hangover
- aloe vera, radish and celery are cooling
- chrysanthemum is an age-old remedy
- onions will get stagnant blood moving
- headaches associated with the common cold will be relieved by eating shallots or thyme
- raw honey when the headache is associated with hypertension
- rye for migraines
- umeboshi plums remove toxins from the body and improve digestion.

Foods to avoid

- those containing tyramine—alcohol, preserved meats, cheese, milk chocolate, soy sauce and yeast—as they make blood pressure rise, causing throbbing headaches or a migraine
- artificial sweeteners and MSG (monosodium glutamate)
- caffeine from all sources—soft drinks, diet pills, cocoa and some painkillers.

Herbal medicine

- feverfew is specific for headaches, including migraines
- liver herbs, such as burdock, dandelion, peppermint, schisandra or St Mary's thistle

- willow bark (the source of aspirin) for pain of any kind
- chamomile or peppermint for headaches associated with digestive trouble
- *Ginkgo biloba* for circulation to the brain
- culinary herbs, such as spearmint and peppermint, which are cooling.

Supplements

- magnesium relaxes muscles—great for tension headaches
- vitamin C for circulation; it also protects against the effects of environmental pollutants and reduces allergic responses
- vitamin E for circulation
- B complex for the nervous system
- spirulina, wheatgrass or chlorella are cooling and will keep your liver and digestion happy
- add chlorophyll to your water.

Lifestyle factors

- maintain good digestive health
- ensure regular bowel movements
- eat regularly
- identify any allergen and avoid it
- get your back checked, as strain may trigger pain
- drink loads of purified water
- manage stress, particularly anger, resentment and frustration
- keep your liver happy by eating plenty of leafy green vegetables and reducing toxins such as processed and refined foods, alcohol, tobacco and animal products
- cut down on your exposure to toxins by using natural cleaning products, and skin- and body care products

- maintain a healthy blood pressure
- eliminate toxic chemicals from your life.

Essential oils

- peppermint, ginger or wintergreen (diluted) rubbed onto the back of your neck
- lavender (diluted) rubbed onto temples for frontal headaches—or try a lavender bath.

See also COLDS AND 'FLU, INFLAMMATORY CONDITIONS and LIVER.

HERBAL TEAS

The first cup moistens my lips and throat;
the second cup breaks my loneliness;
the third cup searches my inmost being...
The fourth cup raises a slight perspiration
—all the wrong of life passes away from my pores.
At the fifth cup I am purified;
the sixth cup calls me to the realms of the immortals.
The seventh cup—ahhhh, but I could take no more!
I feel only the breath of cold wind that rises in my sleeves...

LO-T'UNG
CHINESE POET, T'ANG DYNASTY

For centuries herbs have been valued for their incredible versatility, being used as medicine, perfumes, foods, in religious ceremonies and as simple teas. It may come as a surprise that herbs, the oldest form of medicine on our planet, are still used as the primary form of curative measure by more than 75 per cent of the world's population. While a skilled medical herbalist will conduct a consultation to assess your overall health in terms of diet, lifestyle, emotional factors and other body relationships before prescribing a specific treatment, even the simplest of herbal teas available off the shelf are able to energise, relax, restore, revitalise and assist in improving your metabolic functioning. It's not just the therapeutic properties of the herbs that make you feel better; the whole idea of preparing a herbal tea, with its rich aromas and colours, along with the ritual of sitting and drinking with friends, or by yourself, will reduce the stress of 'life'.

How to prepare

Baths Steep 200 grams of dried herbs in cold water for twelve hours, then heat the infusion, strain into the bath water and lie back and relax in the bath for ten to fifteen minutes.

Decoctions Primarily used for hard or woody plant materials such as roots, barks and seeds—place one heaped teaspoon of herbs per cup of cold water in a saucepan, bring to the boil, simmer (covered) for ten to fifteen minutes, then strain.

Infusions To brew a pot of herbal tea, pour boiled water over the herbs (use one heaped teaspoon of dried herb per cup of water) and allow to steep (two to three minutes for plant leaves, five minutes for flowers), then strain; or use a tea infuser.

Poultices In a saucepan, bring water to the boil, insert a sieve containing fresh or dried herbs, cover and steam for a few minutes, remove the sieve and drain the herbs, then spread the softened, warm herbs on a woollen cloth and place on the affected area for two hours.

Blends

Brain power Sage, rosehips, damiana and lemonbalm.

Colds and 'flu Yarrow, elderflower, mullein, calendula, thyme and peppermint.

Detox Red clover, calendula, peppermint, burdock and schisandra.

Digestive aid Chamomile, peppermint and meadowsweet.

Gut soother Licorice root, marshmallow root and slippery elm.

Hormone balance Wild yam, licorice, dong quai and red clover.

Mood elevator Lavender, damiana, St John's wort and lemonbalm.

Pick-me-up (mental and physical) Siberian ginseng, sage, rosehips, lemonbalm, damiana and tulsi

Post-party Pau d'arco, peppermint, skullcap, lemonbalm and St John's wort.

Sleep Chamomile, lemonbalm, skullcap and valerian.

HERPES

There are two types of herpes—herpes simplex virus (HSV) 1 and 2. The first one causes cold sores and sometimes inflammation of the cornea of the eye. Approximately 80 per cent of the population are infected with this virus without symptoms, but about 10 to 20 per cent do experience symptoms. HSV2 causes genital herpes. Both HSV1 and HSV2 are highly contagious.

Herpes is a virus that remains in the body (it lives in nerve cells, where immune cells can't find it) and may lie dormant until there is a trigger, which could be a fever (heat), another viral infection such as a cold or 'flu, exposure to too much sun or wind, stress, menstruation or low immunity. Oral sex can spread the virus from one part to another. The good news is that outbreaks rarely appear after the age of 50.

The symptoms usually consist of tenderness in the affected area (lip, for example, in the case of HSV1) followed by tingling, burning, then blisters. There can also be localised pain, fever, headaches and 'flu-like symptoms. Pus may ooze from the affected area once the painful ulcers erupt, then the blisters crust over and dry when healing. HSV1 will appear two to seven days after exposure and affect the mouth, lips or eyes and lymph nodes.

In women, HSV2 blisters will appear around the rectum, clitoris, cervix and vagina four to eight days after exposure. Women may experience a watery discharge from the urethra and pain when urinating. A pregnant woman with an outbreak near her due date puts her baby at risk of blindness, brain damage and possibly death if she delivers naturally, so a caesarean is usually recommended if this occurs. Men will have a breakout of blisters on the penis, groin and scrotum, again four to eight days after exposure. They also experience a urethral discharge and pain when urinating. Swelling of the penis and foreskin is also possible. Swollen lymph nodes in the groin may result. In severe cases HSV can cause liver inflammation.

Helpful foods

- lysine, an amino acid found in fish, is essential—the balance between lysine and arginine (see page 134) needs to be controlled so supplementation is usually necessary
- essential fatty acids—found in flaxseed oil, chia seeds, spirulina and olive oil—are important for skin healing
- shiitake mushrooms are antiviral and immune-boosting
- sulfur in spinach relieves irritation and is high in vitamin A
- dulse, a sea vegetable, is an old remedy for HSV.

Foods to avoid

- junk, processed and refined foods
- sugar
- tomatoes, citrus fruits and juices when you experience an outbreak
- those high in arginine—milk chocolate, nuts, soy, spinach, lentils, crustaceans, eggs, wheat, soy and red meat.

Herbal medicine

- echinacea for immunity
- golden seal for wound healing
- St John's wort as an antiviral, anti-inflammatory and antidepressant—at the first sign of an outbreak, use diluted St John's wort topically
- echinacea, myrrh and tea tree oil diluted and applied topically for their antiseptic properties
- licorice reduces the effects of cell damage and inhibits growth.

Supplements

- lysine fights the virus and reduces arginine—an amino acid that plays an important role in the formation of white blood cells, which are vital for immunity—therefore it is recommended you stay on a lysine supplement for no longer than six months
- vitamin B to reduce stress and improve gut flora
- zinc for wound healing, immunity and skin—zinc lozenges will help keep your mouth healthy
- garlic for its antibacterial properties
- vitamin C for immunity and wound healing
- vitamin A prevents infection spreading, is healing and can be applied topically.

Lifestyle factors

- if you suffer from regular outbreaks, consider having your thyroid checked
- allergies will make you more susceptible
- avoid heat in any form
- avoid smoking and alcohol
- reduce stress
- ice packs are very helpful, especially at the first sign of an outbreak
- keep lesions dry
- take a bath in bancha tea or make a strong tea, soak a cloth in it and apply topically; perhaps add a drop of both tea tree and lavender oils
- maintain good genital hygiene
- wear only cotton underwear and change it daily—more often if there is a discharge.

See also Bancha tea, Colds and 'flu, Fever, Immunity, Sea vegetables and Stress.

Essential oils

🌿 diluted lavender oil (1 drop in ½ cup water), topically.

HIV AND AIDS

HIV (human immunodeficiency virus), the virus that causes AIDS (acquired immune deficiency syndrome), attacks your immune cells, the T lymphocytes. This causes a breakdown of your immunity, which is why keeping the health of your immune system at optimum level is of vital importance. Deaths occur not from AIDS, but because of one of the many infections or cancers that invade a compromised body, made possible by decreased immunity. Like other retroviruses spread through sexual contact or blood, through shared intravenous drug use or blood transfusions, HIV can remain unnoticed in your body for years.

If your immune system is kept in good order, then chances are you may never contract AIDS, even if you have HIV. Many people live relatively healthy lives with HIV, and in my experience they become healthier than they were before due to their newfound vigilance. It is estimated only 15 to 20 per cent of those with HIV go on to develop the more severe symptoms categorised as AIDS. Those at risk have lowered immunity, are IV drug users, are promiscuous, usually young males, and men who have unprotected sex with men.

In the weeks following exposure some people may experience mild 'flu-like symptoms as the body starts to produce antibodies against the virus. However, HIV symptoms don't usually appear for two to five years. Symptoms include fatigue, diarrhoea, weight and appetite loss, enlarged lymph nodes, night sweats, inflammation in the mouth and gums, skin problems and enlarged liver and/or spleen. Oral thrush, indicated by white lumps on the tongue, is a common sign. Pneumonia, Epstein-Barr virus, cytomegalovirus and herpes simplex viruses are common, as is tuberculosis. Diagnosis is made through a blood test looking for HIV antibodies.

Helpful foods

- those high in vitamin A, such as yellow, green, orange and red fruit and vegetables
- those that aid the liver, such as cabbage, broccoli, brussels sprouts and kale
- lots of fresh juices (with garlic if you can tolerate it), including carrot, beetroot, kale and spinach
- wheatgrass every day, either juiced or as a supplement—you can take up to 100 millilitres a day
- shiitake mushrooms for immune-boosting and antiviral properties
- high-fibre foods such as fruit and vegetables, chia seeds, LSA and wholegrains
- quality plant protein is essential for keeping your weight at a healthy level
- umeboshi plums for so many reasons
- turmeric as an anti-inflammatory and for its positive effect on the liver.

Foods to avoid

- animal products are to be eaten sparingly only, if at all—if you must eat them, make sure you buy organic produce
- limit unfermented soy products, but don't eliminate them
- all processed and refined foods
- sugar and saturated fats
- yeast
- try to pinpoint foods you are sensitive to and eliminate them from your diet.

Herbal medicine

- phyllanthus, gotu kola and olive leaf are great antiviral herbs
- immune-boosting astragalus will help nutrient assimilation
- aloe vera appears to inhibit the growth and spread of HIV—it will also soothe your gut lining
- echinacea (use the whole plant) is blood-cleansing and a strong immune booster
- cat's claw and andrographis are also great immune boosters
- liver herbs are very important—use ones such as schisandra, St Mary's thistle, andrographis, burdock, licorice and dandelion root
- golden seal is helpful as it cleanses the blood and lymphatic system, and is good for viral and bacterial infections, to boost immunity and to reduce inflammation in mucous membranes
- pau d'arco is important for its immune-boosting, antifungal, antibiotic and antioxidant properties
- digestive herbs such as chamomile, peppermint, gentian, andrographis, meadowsweet and astragalus
- for nausea, try peppermint, ginger, chamomile or raspberry leaf tea
- grapeseed extract is a strong antioxidant.

Note: Due to drug interaction, St John's wort is contraindicated for those on HIV medication.

Supplements

- acidophilus to supply essential 'good' bacteria to the intestinal tract and liver—candida is strongly associated with HIV
- antioxidants such as vitamins A and C, coenzyme Q10
- coenzyme Q10 for circulation, energy to improve immunity and the health of the heart as well
- selenium to fight free radicals and increase immunity

- slippery elm balances water in the colon, so it is helpful in reducing diarrhoea—it also coats the digestive tract from top to bottom, so it will help with any digestive complaint
- B vitamins for the gut, nervous system and brain function—consider an injection from your GP
- amino acids supply protein, so they will repair and rebuild tissues
- garlic will be helpful due to its antibiotic, immuno-stimulant and digestive properties—it is also helpful in combating candida
- chlorella will help repair tissues and build up immunity—it is also antiviral and will improve liver health
- choline from soy lecithin is helpful for inhibiting the growth of lymphoid cells
- immune-boosting vitamin A helps with the health of your heart and also fights free radicals; it may have anti-cancer properties, and it will fight infection and increase your longevity
- quercetin in green tea and vitamin C helps prevent allergic reactions and increase immunity; quercetin also inhibits retroviruses
- essential fatty acids from flaxseed or fish oils, evening primrose and olive oils, or just flaxseed—some patients swear by fish oil to help reduce sunken cheeks
- shiitake, reishi and maitake mushrooms are available in a liquid form and have very strong immune-boosting, antiviral and anti-cancer properties—maitake has been seen to kill HIV in the laboratory
- digestive enzymes will most likely be needed
- fibre from slippery elm, oat bran and psyllium husks—be sure to follow with a glass or two of water
- royal jelly or propolis will be helpful for bacterial infections and immunity; check for allergy.

Lifestyle factors

- always use a condom with a spermicide when there is any sexual contact
- seek out the advice and guidance of a qualified natural health practitioner along with that of your GP—make sure both are educated and knowledgeable on the latest HIV/AIDS treatments and drug interactions
- HIV drugs have many side effects—consult your naturopath about the best ways to reduce symptoms. You don't need more drugs to combat the effect of the others, so where you can go natural, do so
- treatments such as massage, acupuncture, kinesiology and counselling will be of great benefit
- don't see a diagnosis of HIV as a death sentence, it isn't—it is a wake-up call from your immune system and spirit; there are people out there, once diagnosed with HIV, who are 'antibody-negative'—surprising but true
- reduce stress
- get enough quality sleep
- it is *very* important to maintain a healthy, highly nutritious diet—a higher than normal intake of nutrients is required due to malabsorption
- as much as possible reduce the burden on your liver by using natural cleaning products and hair- and skincare products, eliminating tobacco, reducing alcohol and avoiding recreational drugs, as they are very hard on your liver, gut, immune system, spirit and brain
- drink purified water only.

See also CANDIDA, DIGESTION, IMMUNITY, PROTEIN, SOY PRODUCTS, UMEBOSHI PRODUCTS and WATER.

HIVES
Refer to IMMUNITY, INFLAMMATORY CONDITIONS and LIVER.

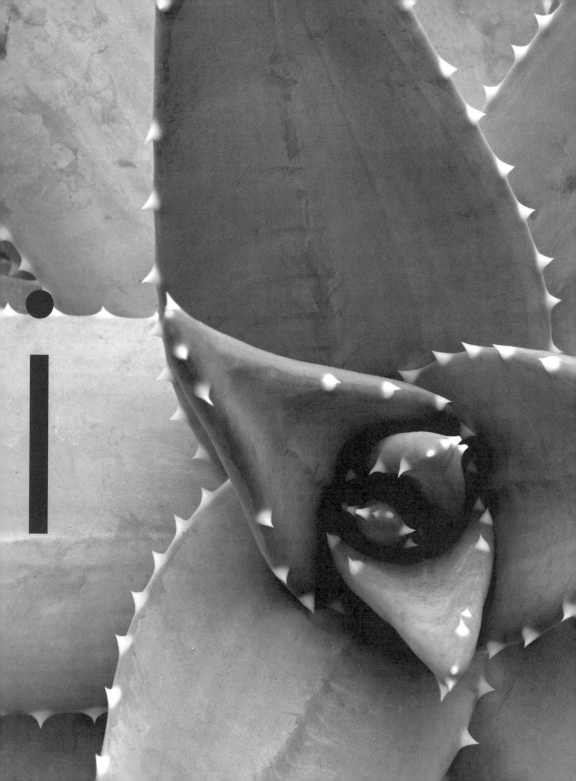

IMMUNITY

Early this century severe acute respiratory syndrome (SARS) caused much panic and the realisation that the rapid development of new infections, especially viruses, is a reality, just another reason to ensure your immune system is able to ward off such conditions. There are two types of virus—enveloped (the virus has an outer coating) and non-enveloped. Although conventional medical treatment has tried antibiotics, antivirals and antibodies, there is still no accepted and effective treatment for dealing with either new viruses or some of the older ones. Herbal medicine can play an important role, not only as a preventative but also in minimising the threat to your health after an infection.

Helpful foods

- umeboshi plums for cold and 'flu-like symptoms, nausea and digestive complaints
- gomashio, a Japanese condiment made by grinding roasted sesame seeds and sea salt together, increases natural immunity and helps prevent disease—it is available in health food stores and Asian supermarkets or you can make your own
- daikon (white radish) or turnip—these were the foods used as medicine during the initial outbreak of SARS in Hong Kong, probably due to their antiviral properties
- shiitake mushrooms are especially strong immune boosters and antivirals
- mushrooms (button) improve immunity against disease-producing micro-organisms
- garlic is a great immune booster and antiviral
- pearl barley
- fresh fruit and vegetables, especially yellow, green, orange and red—these are high in vitamin A, which enhances immunity
- spelt, a wholegrain with a great capacity for strengthening immunity.

Herbal medicine

- immune boosters include echinacea (root only in high doses) and andrographis, which works well with echinacea
- febrifuge for fevers, yarrow, peppermint, chamomile, elder flowers and lime flowers
- respiratory tonics for healthy lung function and coughs include marshmallow root, pleurisy root, white horehound, licorice and thyme
- good antivirals for enveloped viruses are St John's wort, gotu kola, lavender, phyllanthus and cat's claw.

Supplements

- vitamin C may be the most important
- chlorella, spirulina and wheatgrass help the body utilise immune-strengthening nutrients
- vitamin E improves immunity
- zinc is an important immune booster.

Lifestyle factors

- reduce smoking
- reduce your intake of alcohol
- get adequate rest, fresh air and exercise
- eat organic food
- reduce stress and deal with underlying emotional issues
- avoid drinking tap water.

See also Colds and 'flu, HIV and AIDS, and Sesame seeds (for gomashio recipe).

INFLAMMATORY CONDITIONS

Most inflammatory conditions—including arthritis, asthma, eczema, dermatitis, hayfever, hives, irritable bowel syndrome, migraines and sinusitis—are somewhat genetic; they are atopic genes usually passed on from one generation to another. Just because one has this gene, however, doesn't mean the symptoms are unavoidable. It's all about maintaining the good health of your liver and your immune and nervous systems.

Helpful foods

- anti-inflammatory foods such as flaxseed oil; ginger; goats milk; chlorophyll from green vegetables and parsley; olive oil; macadamia nuts; green tea; oily fish such as cod, sustainably caught salmon, mackerel, anchovies and sardines; turmeric; and organic soy products.

Foods to avoid

- inflammatory and acidic foods such as red meat, dairy products, refined wheat (white bread and pasta) and the Nightshade family of vegetables—these are white potatoes, capsicum, eggplant, tomatoes and chillies (the effect of the Nightshade family is neutralised somewhat by cooking with salt or miso; red potatoes have the mildest effect)
- white sugar and salt
- refined fats and fried foods
- processed and junk foods
- acidic substances, such as alcohol, too much raw garlic and coffee
- reduce citrus fruit
- a lot of people also react badly to peanuts, so check for allergy.

Herbal medicine

- anti-allergics such as baical skullcap and albizia
- immune boosters such as echinacea (check for allergic reaction first)
- pau d'arco is antifungal and immune-boosting, and cat's claw and echinacea are immune-boosting
- chickweed applied topically (available as an ointment) for itchiness

- golden seal and mullein to reduce inflammation and irritation—for hayfever, gargle with golden seal if the throat is itchy
- nettle tea cleanses the blood
- gotu kola as an antifungal and antibacterial, and good for skin irritation
- liver herbs such as St Mary's thistle, schisandra or dandelion root are good
- andrographis is fabulous, as it is a liver, digestive and immune herb
- schisandra is used for detoxing the liver and is also great for the symptoms associated with the excesses of modern living
- herbs for your nervous system are essential—try chamomile (also good for digestion), St John's wort (check with your practitioner for drug inter-reactions) and withania (also used to increase energy)
- neem is wonderful for any skin ailment, both internally and externally
- horseradish and turmeric for sinusitis
- blood-cleansing herbs, such as yellow dock, echinacea, dandelion root and burdock—for centuries burdock has been applied topically for any skin problem and taken internally for the liver—will also promote bowel movement
- elder, fenugreek or red clover will loosen the phlegm associated with asthma or sinusitis
- horseradish for hayfever
- ginger and turmeric as anti-inflammatories.

Supplements

- vitamin C with bioflavonoids is essential in cases of inflammation—it will also help the immune system
- blue–green micro-algae such as spirulina, wheatgrass and chlorella
- zinc is important for the skin and immune system
- B complex will help the nervous system

- vitamin E as an antioxidant, immune booster and for improving circulation to the skin
- vitamin A for improved immunity, allergies and skin problems
- omega 3 oils such as flaxseed and chia
- a good probiotic for gut health.

Lifestyle factors

- be sure the bowels move daily
- improve digestion by eating foods that are easy to digest
- avoid the chemicals in cleaning and skincare products, shampoos and conditioners—buy sulfate-free ones—as these chemicals irritate the skin, kidneys, immune system and liver
- sinusitis, if not an allergic reaction, is usually caused by bacteria, smoking, hayfever or an anatomical abnormality—treat the cause first
- keep your liver happy by eliminating the excessive amounts of preservatives and toxins found in conventionally produced fruit and vegetables, cigarettes, alcohol and processed foods
- identify allergens and avoid
- check for food sensitivities and avoid
- viruses or candida can cause hives, so treat the cause first
- antibiotics, aspirin, preservatives, saccharin and eucalyptus, as well as fluoridated water, are likely to create an allergic reaction in those with an atopic gene
- apply aloe vera to hives
- drink purified water only
- your skin is your largest organ, so for extra protection buy a filter for your shower nozzle (available in health food stores), otherwise it will soak up the chlorine and chemicals found in the water supply, aggravating allergies

- topically apply raw honey (manuka is great as it is also antibacterial), umeboshi plums, a rice bran compress or fresh paw paw to hives or eczema
- a nasal douche of warm water and salt is effective against sinusitis
- manage stress by learning a meditation technique or practising yoga
- exposure to the sun and sea has been shown to be beneficial
- moderate and regular exercise is vital
- deal with any underlying, unresolved emotional issues.

See also ARTHRITIS, ASTHMA, ECZEMA, EYES, HEADACHES, IMMUNITY, IRRITABLE BOWEL SYNDROME, LIVER and SKINCARE, NATURAL.

IRIDOLOGY

You can see a lot by looking into someone's eyes. The structure of the fibres, the type and position of the lesions (holes), the colour and many other things can tell us a lot about the person we are looking at.

Different organs hold different emotions and it's sometimes difficult to know which came first—the emotion or the predisposed weakness or strength of the particular organ. Often a predisposition to liver insufficiency is genetic, but it's interesting to note that once again the nature–nurture debate is relevant—that is, if a person has inherited a 'hot' liver and is subjected to the wrong foods and negative emotions, then chances are they will be resentful and have poor digestion, resulting in, for example, nausea, acne or a lack of direction.

Since grief is the emotion attached to the lungs, if you suffer from respiratory problems, chances are there is some unresolved grief, either within you or your genetic line (seven generations back). If you have a child wetting the bed, take a look at what's going on in the kidney area in the iris, as the kidneys store fear and anxiety. (You can use iridology to see 'markers' for such predisposed illnesses in the iris. You can also see your inherited gifts. Incidentally, Western diagnostic methods can't see dysfunction, only pathology.)

Those with open weaves in the iris are more likely to be creative, intuitive and tend towards a weaker constitution. Those with straight fibres that are close together are more analytical and practical and generally have a stronger constitution.

There are only true brown eyes or true blue eyes. Those with hazel or green (and some seemingly brown) eyes are actually blue-eyed with a hereditary layer of accumulated yellow toxicity over the iris. True brown-eyed people are predisposed to liver conditions, such as digestive complaints, skin conditions and allergies, leading to emotional states such as anger and resentment. If you are blue-eyed you are genetically predisposed to inflammatory conditions. This does not mean that if you're brown-eyed, you are exempt—you're not.

You should ensure you get adequate vitamin A and consider the health of your liver. Chinese medicine tells us that the liver controls the eyes and its tendons, so liver health is vital for good eye health.

It is now essential that you learn to *listen* to what your body is trying to tell you. Where you come from genetically is a good start. 'Know thyself.' By first knowing then accepting what car you drive, so to speak, you'll know what you can do with it. A Porsche doesn't like off-road driving, and four-wheel drives don't perform at their peak in the city. Iridology is a great tool for finding out these things, then working with what you've got.

IRON

Many people think that only women suffer from an iron deficiency, and usually only after menstruation. Another misconception is that the only symptom of this mineral deficiency is fatigue. Not so.

Iron is important for digestion, energy, immunity, growth and mental stability. The usual suspects when deficiencies occur are heavy periods, poor digestion, too much coffee and tea, a long-term illness, excessive exercise, heavy sweating, long-term use of antacids, cancer, candida, chronic herpes, rheumatoid arthritis and parasites. There is a long list of physical symptoms including:

anaemia	mental slowness
brittle bones	mouth ulcers and inflammation
brittle hair	muscle spasms
digestive trouble	nails with long ridges or spoon-shaped nails
dry eyes	night sweats
dry skin	pale complexion
fatigue	premature greying
feeling faint	spots in your vision
hair loss	trembling arms or hands
headaches	trouble swallowing
irregular, very light or absent periods	weak tendons
lower back pain	weight gain

Emotional symptoms include nervousness, depression, irritability and anxiety.

The Australian recommended daily allowances are:

Men	19+	7 mg/day
Women	19–54 years	12–16 mg/day
	54+	5–7 mg/day
	Pregnant	22–36 mg/day
Children	1–11 years	6–8 mg/day
	12–18 years	10–13 mg/day

The average vegetarian diet is able to supply twice the minimum daily requirements of iron—it also supplies the body with three times the minimum daily requirement of vitamin C. Studies of the iron content in food show that vegetables, fruit and nuts are much higher in iron content than beef. So you needn't be a meat eater to get your iron.

Food	Milligrams per 100 g
Amaranth	16.0
Dried bean curd (yuba)	11.0
Soybeans	8.4
Almonds	7.4
Sesame seeds	7.1
Lentils and pulses	>6.9
Sea vegetables	6.3
Dried peaches	6.0
Beef	2.0–3.0
Kale	1.5

Helpful foods

- those high in vitamin C as this will increase iron absorption up to 30 per cent; protein and B vitamins also help with absorption
- molasses
- mochi (pounded sweet rice)
- leafy green vegetables, such as broccoli, watercress, parsley, alfalfa, kale and rocket
- legumes, such as lentils, kidney and soybeans
- locally sourced sea vegetables, such as kelp
- fruit, such as dried peaches, raisins, cherries, mulberries, raspberries and Chinese red dates
- tofu
- sustainably caught seafood
- amaranth
- millet
- wholegrains
- pumpkin and beetroot
- coconut milk
- organic raisins
- nuts and seeds, including sesame seeds, almonds, chestnuts and walnuts.

Foods to avoid
🌿 lots of lemons and limes.

Herbal medicine
🌿 burdock

🌿 cayenne

🌿 chamomile

🌿 dandelion

🌿 fennel seed

🌿 lemongrass

🌿 licorice

🌿 paprika

🌿 peppermint

🌿 rosehip

🌿 nettles.

IRRADIATED FOOD

Why do we expose our food to irradiation? Some 50 countries have decided that it is okay to expose our food to ionising radiation in order to destroy micro-organisms, bacteria, viruses or insects that might be present in the food. We also do it to delay the ripening of fruits or the sprouting of vegetables, increase juice yield and improve rehydration.

Basically, irradiation prolongs the shelf life of food by decreasing the chances of spoilage.

Food irradiation acts by damaging the target organism's DNA beyond its ability to repair. Insects either do not survive or become incapable of reproduction while plants cannot continue their natural ripening processes.

The energy density per atomic transition of ionising radiation is very high; it can break apart molecules and induce ionisation, which is not achieved by mere heating. This is the reason for both new effects and new concerns. The food is exposed to ionising radiation, from gamma rays or a high energy electron beam or powerful X-rays. Both X-rays and gamma rays are a form of radiation that shares some characteristics with microwaves, but is of much higher energy and penetration. The rays pass through the food just like microwaves in a microwave oven, but the food doesn't heat up to any significant extent.

The United States Department of Agriculture (USDA) has approved the use of irradiation as an alternative treatment to pesticides for fruits and vegetables that are considered hosts to a number of insect pests. These include fruit flies and weevils. To add to the horror, the US Food and Drug Administration (FDA) has cleared (among a number of others) the treatment of hamburger patties to eliminate the residual risk of contamination by a virulent *E. coli*.

Irradiated food is required to be labelled as such. Most foods from overseas will be irradiated and sometimes in cans, which are made using toxic chemicals such as BPA and pthalates. Yet another reason to eat SLOW—seasonal, local, organic and whole.

IRRITABLE BOWEL SYNDROME

Irritable bowel syndrome (IBS) has become increasingly prevalent over the past decade or so—it is now considered the most common digestive disorder. It may affect the whole of the gut, from mouth to bottom, or just part. Symptoms of IBS are gas, spasms, cramping, discomfort and bloating, followed by alternating bouts of constipation and diarrhoea. This may be accompanied by nausea, reflux, indigestion and food intolerances. Eating seems to trigger the associated pain. The subsequent poor digestion of food will cause malabsorption of nutrients.

For many years, sufferers were misdiagnosed and orthodox medical practitioners were, and still are, prescribing anti-inflammatory drugs and steroids to treat the symptoms. This kind of treatment is ineffective, even dangerous in the long term. The disease needs to be addressed and the symptoms' severity reduced. Most practitioners now agree that the orthodox dietary suggestion—to recommend soft foods lacking fibre as well as dairy and other animal products—exacerbates this and many other diseases. The IBS patient is also often holding their anxiety in the gastrointestinal tract, so treatment needs to consist of a change in diet to one higher in fibre and low in acid/inflammatory foods, along with methods to address the nervous system. The health of the liver and immune system must also be considered in any treatment.

It is no surprise, really, to see this condition as prevalent as it is, considering the amount of inflammatory, processed foods we consume and, conversely, the insufficient amount of anti-inflammatory foods eaten. Inflammatory foods need to be reduced and replaced with anti-inflammatory foods. Stress also needs to be managed, and herbal medicine is very important for a faster, more complete recovery.

Helpful foods

- anti-inflammatory foods such as deep-sea, cold-water fish—sustainably caught cod, salmon, tuna, mackerel, anchovies, trout and sardines
- anti-inflammatory oils such as olive and flaxseed—these protect the intestinal lining
- high-fibre foods such as fruit and vegetables, wholegrains (oats, brown rice, quinoa), legumes and sprouts
- alfalfa, which contains vitamin K, will help rebuild the intestinal walls and is important for proper digestion
- leafy green vegetables—such as rocket, baby or English spinach, radicchio and Asian greens—will aid the liver, thus digestion
- macadamia nuts, avocado, green tea, turmeric and goats milk products are all anti-inflammatory
- miso is wonderful here, as it lines and soothes the gastrointestinal tract

and also helps to balance gut flora—eat lots and be sure to buy miso without MSG that has not been genetically altered (buying organic is the way to go with all soy products).

Foods to avoid

- inflammatory foods, such as red meat, dairy products, refined wheat and sugar and their products
- in severe cases the Nightshade family of vegetables may need to be reduced—these are white potatoes, capsicum, eggplant, tomatoes and chillies—as they also prevent calcium absorption
- fizzy drinks and artificial sweeteners
- all caffeine from milk chocolate, cocoa, drinks and coffee
- processed and refined oils, junk food and intoxicants
- alcohol, tobacco and lactose (from dairy) irritate the stomach lining.

Herbal medicine

- aloe vera to soothe, cleanse and relax the bowel
- digestive herbs, such as meadowsweet, gentian, chamomile and peppermint
- immune-boosting herbs, such as echinacea (also cleanses the blood), andrographis (also good for the liver and digestion), pau d'arco (also antifungal) and astragalus (also helps nutrient absorption)
- herbs for the nervous system, such as chamomile, St John's wort, withania, oats, passionflower and valerian, which is high in magnesium and specific for the gastrointestinal tract nerves
- golden seal, marshmallow and slippery elm coat the gastrointestinal tract by working on inflamed mucous membranes.

Herbal teas

- try chamomile, peppermint, meadowsweet, passionflower and ginger.

Supplements

- fibre from slippery elm, psyllium husks and oat bran—be sure to drink at least one glass of water after taking
- aloe vera
- magnesium for spasms or muscular pains
- vitamin B for muscle tone and the nervous system
- acidophilus to restore healthy gut flora
- flaxseed oil is invaluable here for its high content of essential fatty acids.

Lifestyle factors

- exercise regularly and in moderation—yoga, walking and swimming are very helpful
- identify sources of stress and try to manage them
- chew your food well
- avoid eating late at night
- try to deal with any underlying emotional issues, especially grief and sadness—these emotions are associated with the colon, which is especially sensitive in autumn; let go
- antibiotics, laxatives, antacids and steroids disturb gut flora
- check for candida
- rule out more serious illnesses such as Crohn's disease, ulcerative colitis, colon cancer and diverticulitis
- avoid alcohol, tobacco and recreational drugs.

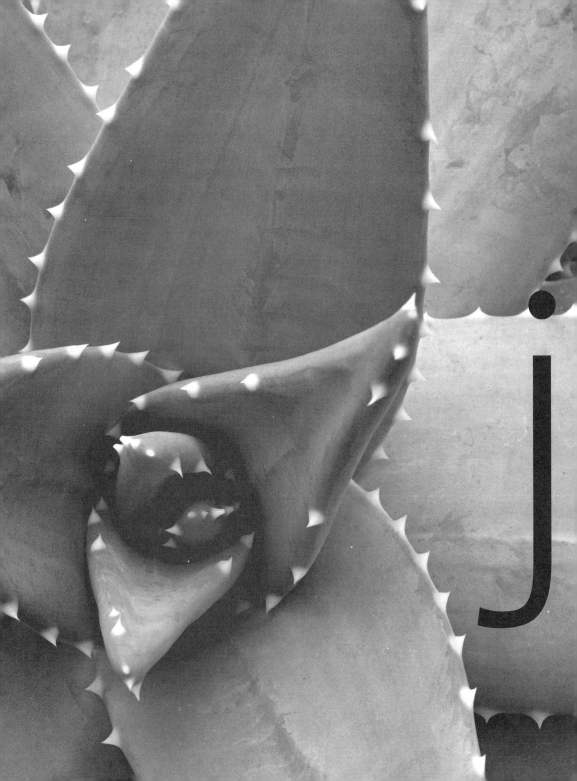

j

JUICES

Consuming fresh fruit and vegetable juices is a very good habit to get into, especially first thing in the morning. They contain an array of vitamins, minerals, enzymes, purified water, proteins, carbohydrates, chlorophyll and various co-factors that enhance individual nutrients. Little digestion is needed for their assimilation, so they are a quick way to restore nutrients to starved cells.

Canned and bottled juices are not as good as fresh juices, as they are usually made from concentrates and not whole foods, nor do they contain live enzymes. Moreover, the liquids from which they are reconstituted may not be of the highest standard, and additives such as sugar, salt, artificial colours and flavours and chemical preservatives are usually added. There are, however, some good packaged juices available (read the label and avoid those with anything added or taken out).

Drink juices at other than meal times or on a empty stomach, as your system digests them much faster than solids. Try the following juices, either on their own or in combination with others, for specific conditions.

When buying a juicer, be sure to get one that has low revolutions per minute. If it zips around really fast, allowing a carrot or apple to be juiced whole, then the enzymes will be destroyed by the heat created by the motor.

Acne Carrot, cucumber, parsnip and wheatgrass.
Ageing Wheatgrass.
Anaemia Alfalfa, beetroot greens, kale, parsley, watercress and wheatgrass.
Arthritis Carrot, cucumber, kale, turnip and wheatgrass.
Asthma Cabbage, carrot, celery, kale, radish, turnip and wheatgrass.
Bladder Cabbage, carrot, parsley, parsnip, fresh tomato, turnip and its greens, watercress and wheatgrass.
Blood pressure regulation Beetroot, cucumber, spinach and wheatgrass.

Blood sugar regulation Artichoke, bean sprout, carrot, kale, parsnip, spinach, turnip and its greens, and wheatgrass.

Bones Alfalfa, carrot, parsnip, fresh tomato and wheatgrass.

Bronchitis Celery, fennel, turnip and wheatgrass.

Cancer Asparagus, beetroot and its greens, carrot, kale, parsley, spinach, turnip and its greens, and wheatgrass.

Circulation, improving Beetroot and its greens, kale, parsley, spinach, turnip and its greens, watercress and wheatgrass.

Colitis Cabbage, spinach and wheatgrass.

Constipation Apple, cabbage, celery, prune, spinach and wheatgrass.

Cough Shallots.

Digestive disorders Ginger, lemon and spinach.

Eczema Cucumber and radish.

Eye disorders Alfalfa, asparagus, beetroot and its greens, parsley, parsnip, turnip and its greens, and wheatgrass.

Fatigue Alfalfa, artichoke, beetroot and its greens, and wheatgrass.

Female hormonal imbalance Parsley and watercress.

Fever Cucumber.

Fluid retention Bean sprouts, cucumber and watermelon.

Gout Asparagus, celery, fennel and fresh tomato.

Hair loss Alfalfa, cabbage, cucumber, kale, watercress and wheatgrass.

Hayfever Carrot, kale, parsnip and wheatgrass.

Heart disease Beetroot and its greens, parsley, shallots, spinach, and turnip and its greens.

Impotence Alfalfa, kale and wheatgrass.

Insomnia Celery and lettuce.

Kidney disorders Alfalfa, asparagus, beetroot and its greens, cabbage, celery and cucumber.

Liver disorders Alfalfa, beetroot and its greens, carrot, celery, kale, parsnip, spinach, tomato, turnip and its greens, watercress and wheatgrass.

Lung disorders Turnip and its greens, and wheatgrass.

Lymphatic circulation Beetroot and its greens, and Swiss chard.

Menopause Beetroot and its greens, and Swiss chard.

Menstrual problems Beetroot and its greens, Swiss chard, watercress, wheatgrass.

Mucus removal Radish and shallots.

Nervous system disorders Asparagus, celery, fennel, lettuce, spinach and wheatgrass.

Pregnancy and labour Alfalfa, bean sprouts, beetroot and its greens, carrot, kale, parsnip and Swiss chard.

Prostate trouble Asparagus and parsley.

Psoriasis Cucumber.

Pyorrhoea Cabbage, kale and spinach.

Rheumatism Asparagus.

Sinusitis Ginger, lemon, radish and wheatgrass.

Skin disorders Asparagus, beetroot and its greens, parsley, parsnip, radish, shallots, spinach, tomato, turnip and its greens, watercress and wheatgrass.

Thyroid disorders Alfalfa, cabbage, radish, spinach and watercress.

Ulcers Cabbage, carrot, kale, parsnip, spinach and wheatgrass.

Urinary tract infection Parsley.

Weight loss Alfalfa, bean sprouts, beetroot and its greens, carrot, celery, cucumber, fennel, parsnip, parsley, radish, shallots, spinach, tomato, turnip and its greens, watercress and wheatgrass.

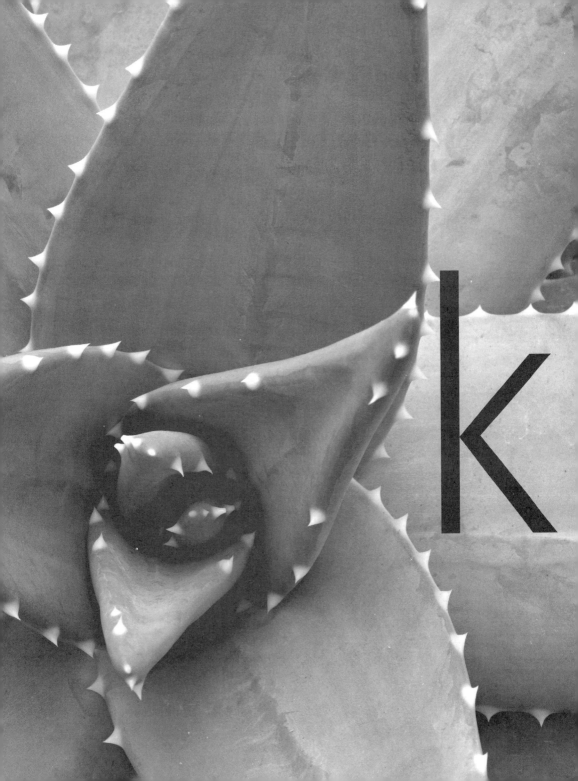

k

KALE

How wonderful we now have kale on our plates, but if you haven't, due to lack of availability, then grow it. Actually, grow it anyway. It's super easy to cultivate and grows well through winter, tasting sweeter and developing more flavour after it's been exposed to frost. Kale is a form of cabbage but the central leaves don't form a head. It is also kind enough to freeze well, so when you have an abundance in the garden, just wash, chop and freeze it.

Kale has more antioxidants than any other vegetable and also a good amount of calcium and iron for its weight. It's also very high in vitamin A (betacarotene), vitamin C and sulforaphane (a chemical with anti-cancer properties). Like its relatives in the Brassica family, it is a source of indole-3-carbinol, which boosts DNA repair in cells and may block the growth of cancer cells.

There are a few different types—curly (Scots kale), plain-leafed, rape and cavolo nero, also called black or Tuscan cabbage. Kale is high in chlorophyll, so we know it's great for the liver. It is also high in fibre, so, when cooked, it's good for the gut, helping it to bind to bile acids, thus removing cholesterol. The antioxidants are helpful in combating free radicals, and kale is super high in vitamin K (so avoid it if you're on blood-thinning medication such as warfarin).

Unlike baby spinach, kale doesn't lose its shape or integrity in cooking, and it's great in stir-fries, soups and smoothies, or added to hummus and dips.

KAMUT

An unadulterated, older variety of cereal from ancient Egypt, the grains of kamut are often three times the size of modern wheat. It is high in protein as well as rich in amino acids and vitamins. It is higher in protein and unsaturated fatty acids than modern wheat, and tastes much better.

As farmers began using hybridised wheat after World War II, kamut almost became extinct. However, a few grains were discovered in a crypt in Egypt and ended up in America—Montana is the home of an abundance of organic wheat such as kamut. Most people with intolerances to wheat have no such reaction to kamut. Available in a flake, flour or the grain, kamut contains gluten, but most of us tolerate it.

See also WHOLEGRAINS.

KELP
Refer to SEA VEGETABLES.

KIDS' LUNCHBOXES
What kids eat during school hours has to be not only nutritious but also able to sustain them for a full day of study. Examples of good choices for morning tea and lunch follow.

Options	Morning tea	Lunch
Example 1	homemade muesli bars or bliss balls (see recipe on page 165) 1 small pear, cut up in a container	mini frittatas fruit juice diluted with water (frozen in summer)
Example 2	yoghurt and chopped fruit in a thermos with sesame seeds, goji berries or chia seeds with organic honey or rice syrup drink (as above)	savoury muffins carrot and celery sticks with a container of pumpkin hummus
Example 3	pan-fried tempeh and sweet potato drizzled with tamari drink (as above)	pumpkin soup and mountain bread organic fruit strap

To keep the different types of food fresh and separate from other food in the lunchbox, you'll need various pieces of equipment. The items you can use include a one cup-sized thermos with a wide mouth (may be used for soups in winter and for fruit and yoghurt in summer); a muffin tin for cooking savoury muffins and mini frittatas; a small icepack to keep lunches cool, especially if you're packing meat or chicken; different sized takeaway containers in non-BPA plastic that fit into lunchboxes—kids love these as you can give them a variety of things in one lunch; a stainless steel double-decker lunch box with smaller containers inside for cut fruit and hummus etc.; and a drink bottle, also in non-BPA plastic.

DO'S AND DON'TS

Do include fruit and/or raw vegetables with every lunch—carrot or celery sticks are good, as are bean shoots and strawberries or other soft fruit.

Don't make fruit and vegetables large, as kids won't eat them, and avoid bananas—they cause phlegm and get squashed. If your child tends to get a runny nose, ear problems, frequent colds or is generally weak, limit fruit intake or include only cooked fruit.

Do include calcium as much as possible.

Don't only supply it from dairy products, if at all (see *Calcium*).

Do include iron-rich foods.

Don't always get it from animal sources.

Do sometimes give them dried fruit.

Don't give them non-organic dried fruit.

Do include protein from vegetable and organic fermented soy products.

Don't give them too many legumes, beans or animal products.

Do make extra soup when making it for the family and freeze it in small containers for lunchboxes.

Don't leave preparing lunches until the morning just before school—the precious time you have in the morning shouldn't be spent preparing food or, worse still, looking for containers and drink bottles.

Do give them an interesting and nourishing morning tea.

Don't make it too large, as this is one way to become an unpopular parent—most schools don't allow the kids to play until their food is finished, so for morning recess, which is about twenty minutes, allow about ten minutes' eating time.

Do include carbohydrates in their lunch.

Don't make it white bread—wholegrains are healthier. Kids don't like large bread rolls either.

Do use wax paper to wrap lunches, where possible. Or, even better, put the food straight into the lunchbox.

Don't always use cling film or aluminium foil.

Do put salad in their sandwiches.

Don't add tomatoes—kids won't eat soggy sandwiches.

Do shop before Monday and buy enough to last the week.

Don't buy pre-packaged foods, unless it is very natural or necessary.

Do give them crackers, such as rice or spelt crackers.

Don't always give them wheat crackers, unless they're spelt.

Do include a drink such as a fruit juice or water—you can freeze it in the non-BPA drink bottle, and in summer it will act as an ice pack.

Don't include milk drinks or by lunchtime they will be spoiled and yucky, unless it's rice milk. Always dilute juice with water, especially for younger children.

Do make finger food as much as possible.

Don't use heavy dressings or saucy things—kids won't eat it if it looks gooey.

Mini corn fritters

These are full of essential nutrients. I've used navy beans in this recipe instead of eggs to bind the ingredients together. Try using other veggies also.

MAKES ABOUT 12 FRITTERS

3 tbsp olive oil or rice bran oil

1 small white onion, diced

1 tbsp finely chopped coriander stems

1 garlic clove, crushed

1 cup corn kernels, cut off the cob

1 cup grated sweet potato

1 zucchini, grated and squeezed dry

1 cup cooked navy beans, rinsed and drained

½ cup finely chopped mint leaves

½ tbsp sea salt, or to taste

2 tbsp brown rice flour or besan

1 lime, quartered

1   In a saucepan, heat 1 tablespoon of the oil and sauté the onion and coriander over medium heat until the onion is translucent. Now add the garlic and stir for a few seconds. Next add the veggies, stir to coat in the oil and sauté for 1 minute until the veggies start to cook. Remove from the heat.

2   Place the navy beans in a bowl and mash with a fork. Add the veggie mixture, mint and salt. Slowly mix in the flour until you have a firm mixture that you can roll into balls. Taste for seasoning. Shape into 12 balls about the size of a walnut, then press into patties.

3   Heat the remaining oil in a large frying pan and fry the fritters, in batches of six to eight, depending on the size of your pan, until golden on each side. Drain on paper towel. Serve with the lime quarters.

Bliss balls (or muesli bars)

MAKES APPROX. 20 BLISS BALLS OR 30 MUESLI BARS

1 cup puffed millet, amaranth, quinoa or brown rice
½ cup desiccated coconut
½ cup sesame seeds
½ cup sunflower seeds
½ cup rice malt
½ cup tahini
1 cup almond meal
1 cup chopped dry roasted nuts (almonds, cashews, brazil, hazelnuts etc.)
     but omit if there are nut allergies
1 cup chopped organic dried apricot, or any other dried fruit

1   Place all the dry ingredients in a food processor and mix together.
    Gradually add the tahini and the rice malt. For bliss bombs, use wet
    hands to roll the mixture into walnut-sized balls, then roll them in
    sesame seeds or the coconut. For muesli bars, press the mixture evenly
    into a lightly oiled (rice bran, macadamia or coconut oil) tray. Before
    baking, slice into small rectangles with a knife that has been held under
    the hot water tap. Bake for 15 to 20 minutes at 180°C. The bars will still
    be soft, so let them cool and harden before breaking them apart.
2   Wrap individual bars in wax paper and freeze, although they'll last
    for months in an airtight container out of the fridge. Pull out before
    school and put into the lunchbox—they will be defrosted by morning
    tea time.

Note: The above measurements are rough as there are no set amounts.
Add more of what your child likes and less of what they don't like. Adjust
sweetness and consistency with tahini and rice malt.

Vegan carrot and zucchini muffins

The tofu holds the muffins together and is great for balancing your blood sugar in the afternoon. The mixture will freeze well too, so make lots and cook as you need them.

MAKES 12

1 cup water
250 g palm sugar or coconut palm sugar
½ tsp each cinnamon, nutmeg and cardamom powder
2½ cups wholewheat spelt flour (or any other flour)
2 tsp each baking powder and bicarbonate of soda
1 cup chopped walnuts
1 tbsp poppy seeds
1 cup pepitas
2 tbsp sunflower seeds
1 cup each carrot and zucchini, grated
180 g Omega spread
300 g silken tofu

1   Boil water, grate in the sugar and add the spices. Dissolve the sugar, then allow to cool completely.
2   Mix together the flour, bicarbonate soda, baking powder, walnuts and seeds.
3   In a separate bowl combine the carrot, zucchini and Omega spread. Beat the tofu with a whisk and add to the water mixture. Pour over the veggies and mix.
4   Make a well in the centre of the flour mixture and pour in the veggie mixture. Gently stir to combine. Place in a greased 12-hole muffin tray and bake at 180°C for 25 to 30 minutes. You'll know they're cooked when you stick a skewer into one and it comes out clean.

MENU IDEAS

Morning tea

- rice crackers (no MSG or additives) and a separate container with hummus or pesto
- boiled egg (let them peel it themselves) and crackers
- celery sticks, cut into finger-sized pieces and filled with a nut butter or quark
- organic fruit straps
- homemade muesli bars (see recipe on page 165)—remember to keep them small
- yoghurt and chopped fruit with sesame seeds and organic honey or rice syrup in a thermos
- small pieces of fruit such as apricots, nectarines or grapes
- packets of organic sultanas and apricots mixed together, which is more interesting than sultanas alone
- tempeh, lightly pan-fried with soy sauce.

Lunch

- soup is nice in winter—make a whole lot, then freeze it in small containers until it's needed. Pull it out of the freezer the night before and warm it in the morning, then pack it in a small thermos to take to school. Include a brown roll or flat bread. Some children like chicken noodle, minestrone or miso soup while others prefer a creamier style, such as pumpkin or potato and leek. A thermos can also be used for red lentil dhal or corn chowder. Blend silken tofu through the soup to make it creamy and protein-packed
- savoury frittatas, made with spelt flour, an organic egg or mashed firm tofu, herbs and a vegetable, such as grated zucchini or sautéed mushrooms; brown rice and quinoa are good here also

- ✿ mini pizzas—you can use a bought base such as mountain bread, an organic flat bread or an organic rye pita bread, cut into rounds and topped with homemade tomato sauce and mashed firm tofu or tempeh and pesto. Make a lot and freeze individually in wax paper; they will thaw in the lunchbox
- ✿ flat bread (preferably wheat-free)—wrapped around hummus, salad and avocado, or salad and organic egg, perhaps with some pan-fried tempeh—cut the wraps in half and pop into the box
- ✿ bean salad, which goes nicely in one of those TV-dinner style lunchboxes—you can buy organic beans such as cannellini and chickpeas in non-BPA cans and mix them with some chopped parsley and mint, or stir through a nice sauce such as tomato, puréed roasted pumpkin or pesto, or any diced roast vegetable
- ✿ marinated tofu (you can buy this already done if you like), cut into strips with a tub of hummus and corn thins or spelt crackers
- ✿ mini corn fritters.

KOMBU
Refer to SEA VEGETABLES.

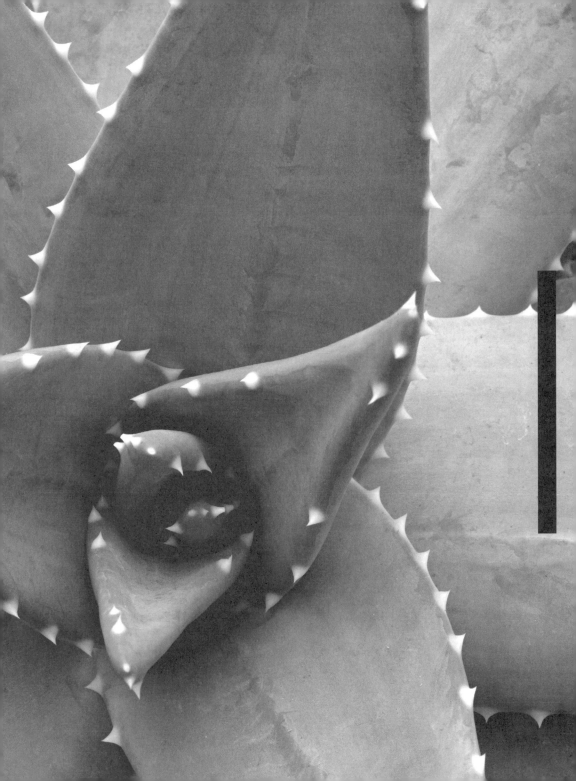

LACTATION

Breastfeeding is a special time for both mother and child. Of course, it doesn't always go to plan. If your baby doesn't latch on or you have decided not to breastfeed, goats milk is the recommended substitute and even this causes a reaction in some little bodies. Please avoid formulas unless they are made from goats milk. Cows milk shouldn't be introduced before twelve months at the earliest. Sometimes you may struggle with your milk flow; the information below will help promote the flow of your milk.

Babies tend to wean themselves, although some never seem to want breastfeeding to stop. The time to start weaning is when they start to show an interest in food—that is, by watching you eat, grabbing for food, or when the 'protrusion reflex' (when the baby stops sticking their tongue out, as they do when breastfeeding) is reduced. If you give them solids before they are ready, they will usually spit them out. They gain cognitive (conscious) control over this, generally at about four to six months of age.

Helpful foods
- lettuce, leafy green vegetables, adzuki beans, black sesame seeds, carrots, soybeans, mochi, avocado, fennel and sweet potato.

Herbal medicine
- burdock, dandelion, ginger and nettle will enrich the milk
- alfalfa, horsetail, raspberry leaf, fennel and *Vitex agnus-castus* (chaste tree) will also help
- try nettle, ginger, fennel, alfalfa or dandelion as a tea.

Supplements
- folic acid
- vitamin B12.

See also BABY, NUTRITION; MASTITIS; and PREGNANCY.

LIVER

A stagnant liver, which in many cases is caused by over-eating or excessive drinking, or by too much stress, means your 'qi' is blocked, causing feelings of sluggishness. This leads to anger and frustration and a sense of being held back. At first when the liver qi becomes blocked you can become depressed or frustrated, then when the qi pushes through the blockage all at once, it shows up as anger. In a physical sense, liver stagnation can cause a sensation of having a lump in the throat or neck or distension in the breasts or abdomen.

Emotionally you may feel repressed, angry, frustrated, resentful, impatient, edgy, depressed, moody or impulsive, make poor judgments, have difficulty making decisions, and experience mental rigidity and negativity. Physically you may suffer allergies, lumps or swelling, chronic indigestion, neck and back tension, fatigue, an inflexible body, eye problems, skin disorders, fingernail or toenail problems, muscular pain, tendon problems and be slow to get going in the morning. Digestive complaints, especially nausea, and reproductive issues may arise. So you can see how vital a healthy liver is for your wellbeing.

Helpful foods

- both pungent and unrefined sweet foods to reduce stagnation
- sour foods, introduced gradually, may also be important, especially if the liver is not only overworked but also weak—lemon juice in warm water in the morning kick starts a sluggish liver, and grapefruit, rye or chamomile will also help
- if you are nervous or agitated, add shallots to your meal for calmness
- cabbage, broccoli and leafy green vegetables promote the digestion of meat.

Foods to avoid

- anything heavy, such as oily or rich food
- processed and refined foods such as white wheat and sugar
- junk food
- all preservatives and chemicals.

Lifestyle factors

- stress headaches are connected to the function of the liver—they may be reduced or eliminated by drinking spearmint tea or eating celery
- anger in the liver can cause insomnia, the type where you can't stop working things over and over in your mind, not even long enough to close your eyes.

See also HEADACHES, SLEEP and SPRING.

A LIVER-FRIENDLY MENU

First thing in the morning, squeeze half a lemon into warm water and drink.

Breakfast—choose one

1 kamut, amaranth or spelt cereal with coconut water or quinoa or rice milk, topped with papaya or another seasonal fruit and chia seeds
2 smoothie with coconut water or rice milk with one teaspoon each of chia seeds, psyllium husks, spirulina, wheat or barley grass as well as fruit such as blueberries and/or paw paw.

Snack—choose one

1 one 200 millilitre glass of fresh carrot, celery, kale, ginger and beetroot juice
2 two corn thins with hummus
3 one cup of sugar-free yoghurt with one teaspoon each of chia seeds, flax meal and raw honey or maple syrup and seasonal fruit
4 smoothie (as above).

Lunch—choose one

1 sandwich or wrap using mountain bread or spelt, kamut or rye sourdough filled with salmon or marinated tofu, avocado, hummus or tahini dressing and salad, such as grated beetroot and carrot, alfalfa and cucumber
2 stir-fried vegetables with tofu (or organic chicken) and brown rice or quinoa, tamari and sesame oil and loads of herbs and leafy greens
3 roast vegetables, cannellini beans and quinoa salad with a little flaxseed oil, vinegar and seasoning
4 big salad with watercress, smoked salmon or legumes, avocado, red cabbage, carrot and any other vegetables you like. Dress with lemon juice, honey and flaxseed or olive oil and serve with a grain or quinoa
5 vegetable frittata.

Snack—choose one

1 bliss balls (see recipe on page 165 under *Kids' lunchboxes*)
2 fresh fruit or vegetable juice
3 three corn thins or spelt crackers with goats cheese, basil, sprouts and pepper or hummus
4 two squares of raw dark chocolate.

Dinner—choose one

1 steamed silken tofu (or organic chicken) with tamari, sesame oil and fish sauce served with steamed vegetables and quinoa
2 baked whole fish with rocket, orange and raddichio salad.

Dessert—choose one

1 yoghurt with fruit and maple syrup, chia seeds and/or flax meal
2 one bliss ball (see recipe on page 165 under *Kids' lunchboxes*)
3 ten dark chocolate-coated goji berries
4 rice milk or coconut water smoothie.

Notes

- drink herbal tea if you like—one teaspoon of raw honey a day is fine
- one to two pieces of fruit a day is enough
- eat your grains during the day.

You need to be nice to your liver because, according to traditional Chinese medicine, the liver stores anger and resentment. In fact, all your organs store different emotions—for example, the kidneys control fear and the lungs grief. Keep your organs happy and they'll take care of your emotions. Keep your mind happy with the right food, exercise and thought patterns and it will take care of your organs.

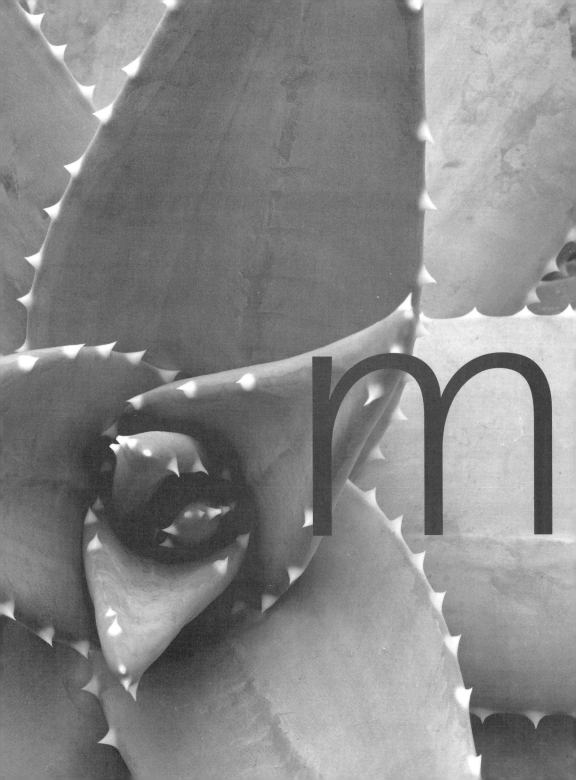

MACA

Maca is a dehydrated root vegetable in the Brassica family grown only in Peru. It resembles a turnip and is a rich source of amino acids, complex carbohydrates, fatty acids and vitamins B, C and E. It has been used by the Peruvians as a medicine and restorative food for more than 5000 years, and has been traditionally used to treat hormonal imbalance, including PMT and menstrual symptoms, osteoporosis, blood sugar imbalance and candida overgrowth, sexual dysfunction and menstrual dysfunction, and for increased endurance (athletes love it). Anti-ageing, it also treats fatigue, both chronic and short term, infertility and decreased libido. Maca is good during convalescence.

It is cultivated by hand at about 4200 metres, free of chemicals and pesticides. The altitude at which it is grown contributes towards its potency.

MAGNESIUM

This essential mineral is important for cardiovascular health, pulling calcium into your bones, good digestion and your nervous system. Low magnesium levels make almost every disease worse. Magnesium is depleted by diarrhoea, diuretics, alcohol, smoking, stress, fluoride, too much protein, drugs (prescription and recreation), silver beet, tea and rhubarb. Signs of deficiency include premenstrual tension, muscle weakness, depression, twitches and cramps, nervousness, irritability, osteoporosis, high cholesterol, insomnia, poor digestion, rapid heart beat, seizures, hypertension, asthma, chronic fatigue, irritable bowel syndrome and dizziness, among others.

Helpful foods

- raw cacao powder
- dried locally sourced sea vegetables
- local beans, such as organic soybeans, mung, black and lima
- wholegrains, such as buckwheat, corn, millet, barley, rye and rice

- nuts and seeds, such as almonds, cashews and sesame seeds
- spirulina and wheatgrass
- leafy dark green vegetables
- sustainably caught fish and other seafood
- peaches
- tofu and tempeh.

See also CALCIUM, CARDIOVASCULAR HEALTH, CRAMPS AND SPASMS, DIGESTION and NUTRIENTS IN FOOD.

MASTITIS

This painful condition occurs when a milk duct in a lactating woman's breast becomes blocked. If it is left untreated, soreness and redness result. 'Flu-like symptoms also appear. In more severe cases an infection may occur.

Try to keep feeding your baby, as the sucking will prevent your breasts getting very full and making the problem worse—feed your baby regularly, offering the least sore side first. Be sure to keep your fluid up and, of course, try to get adequate rest. If pain or symptoms are severe, consult your healthcare practitioner—it may be due to candida. Also try the following:

- if your nipples are cracked and sore, apply aloe vera gel topically, or try flaxseed or chia seed oil for its omega 3 anti-inflammatory properties
- steamed cabbage leaves over the breast have been shown to be very helpful
- between feeds, keep your breasts dry, and try to get some sun on them
- avoid soap and soap-based products, petroleum or alcohol-based products
- try gently massaging your breasts, from the outer circumference towards the nipples
- consider taking some echinacea to boost your immunity.

See also LACTATION.

MEMORY

Most of us expect our ability to remember to deteriorate with age. This is not true, and age has nothing to do with your powers of recall. Neurotransmitters (brain chemicals) are responsible for sending messages around the body, so they are subsequently responsible for bodily functions. If your mind goes blank in the middle of a sentence, it is probable that one of those chemicals has short-circuited, most likely due to an inadequate amount of nutrients supplying them. So sufficient nutrients to the brain are vital for retaining memory through to old age, which is indeed achievable.

Bad fats, such as those from animal fats and processed oils, make your blood more viscous or sticky, thus preventing the blood from flowing smoothly to the brain. Free radicals are dangerous for memory while the B vitamins and amino acids are very important. Alcohol and drugs can cause 'blackouts'. Other contributing factors that cause a negative impact on the brain are allergies, low blood sugar, candida, stress and thyroid imbalance.

Another factor to consider for good brain function is the heart–mind balance. According to traditional Chinese medicine, the heart controls sleep, memory, consciousness, spirit and where the mind is situated. Those with a good balance between their heart and mind often see through problems and arrive at solutions with ease. Their minds are sharp, so take care of the health of your heart, physically and emotionally.

Helpful foods

- foods high in B vitamins, such as brown rice, legumes, nuts, soybeans, tofu and other wholegrains
- sustainably caught fish—vital brain food
- some raw foods eaten each day (less during cooler months).

Foods to avoid

- refined carbohydrates (white flour, white rice)
- refined sugar (white) and its products 'shut down' the brain—it weakens the mind, causing loss of memory and concentration.

Herbal medicine

- *Ginkgo biloba* increases blood flow to the brain
- rosemary is a stimulant, so it is good for recall (a student's best friend)
- basil is good for memory, probably because it increases the circulation of blood
- Siberian ginseng is a stimulant, aiding circulation to the brain; avoid in cases of heart disease or disorders
- brahmi (bacopa) is good for recall.

Supplements

- manganese nourishes the brain and neurotransmitters
- vitamin B complex, particularly B12 for memory, aids neurotransmitters
- vitamin C will help with circulation and allergies
- vitamin E will improve blood flow to the brain
- zinc will bind and remove toxic substances from the brain
- bee pollen (check you are not allergic) contains essential nutrients, including B vitamins and enzymes
- choline (from soy lecithin) is important for neurotransmitter functioning.

Lifestyle factors

- pay attention to what is being said and going on around you, as sometimes as we age our desire to remember decreases
- practise recall
- hold your breath for 30 seconds each day for a month—this will help with mental alertness

- improve poor digestion as this may cause a feeling of heaviness in the head
- parasites may cause memory loss or brain fog
- exercise regularly and moderately
- decrease your free radical load but take synthetic chemicals out of your daily life as much as possible; 'go green' with your cleaning and body products and other household items.

See also BLOOD SUGAR, CANDIDA, CARDIOVASCULAR HEALTH, STRESS and THYROID.

MENOPAUSE

This can begin any time in a woman's life after 35 years of age, but usually the symptoms appear around the ages of 45 to 50 and last for approximately five years. Each woman's attitude towards this 'change of life' will largely determine the severity of the symptoms. Menopause is a natural part of life, not a disease or a punishment.

The symptoms are due to a decrease in the amount of hormones— oestrogen and progesterone—produced by the ovaries. Decreased oestrogen, in particular, is of concern, as it has been linked to cardiovascular disease and osteoporosis. Once thought of as only a sex hormone, we now know that oestrogen receptors are found in the bladder, breasts, arteries, heart, liver, bones, vagina, brain and skin. It is also necessary for maintaining proper functioning of your body's thermostat, to keep the skin in good condition and for proper bone formation.

As the symptoms of menopause can often be unpleasant, it is recommended that they are not ignored. Symptoms include:

bladder problems	dizziness
breast tenderness	dry and ageing skin
depression	dry or itchy vagina
discomfort during intercourse	fatigue

frequent bruising	mood swings
headaches	night sweats
heart palpitations	nose bleeds
hot flushes	poor libido
insomnia	shortness of breath
leg cramps	varicose veins

For controlling the symptoms, a woman has a number of choices. Hormone replacement therapy (HRT), recommended to many women, appears to be of some benefit, but a woman should not make this decision without careful consideration and enquiry. Once you are on HRT, it is recommended you stay on it for life so the symptoms don't reappear. Natural remedies are often a better option than HRT. With the right natural practitioner prescribing you the correct herbal medicine and supplementations, along with exercise and positive thought patterns, there is no need for this to be an unwelcome or annoying time in a woman's life.

Helpful foods

- those high in plant oestrogen
- complex carbohydrates such as fruit and vegetables; grains and seeds such as quinoa, kamut, spelt and brown rice; legumes and nuts and seeds—all these foods are slow to be absorbed in the bloodstream, thus they stabilise blood sugar
- calcium-rich foods (see *Calcium*)
- magnesium-rich foods (see *Magnesium*)
- good oils, such as those found in fish, flaxseed, chia seed, coconut, safflower or olive, will help to lubricate the vagina
- beetroot eaten with carrots.

Foods to avoid

- those that make the blood more acidic, as this increases hot flushes and releases calcium from your bones

- beet greens, plums, cranberry and spinach are high in oxalic acid, which inhibits calcium absorption.

Herbal medicine

- oestrogenic herbs are very important—black cohosh, fennel, sage, unicorn root, raspberry and wild yam root
- herbs that will decrease hot flushes are sage, zizyphus and dong quai
- *Vitex agnus-castus* (chaste tree) is extremely beneficial, as it balances the body's natural levels of progesterone and oestrogen—2.5 millilitres should be taken once a day upon rising
- for mood swings try St John's wort (check for drug interactions), damiana (also used to increase sexual desire and pleasure), withania (also good for increasing energy) and motherwort (also a heart tonic)
- valerian root, chamomile, skullcap and passionflower will promote a restful sleep.

Supplements

- lecithin granules will reduce flushes and other symptoms
- evening primrose oil and vitamin E will help reduce hot flushes and are important for the production of oestrogen
- calcium and magnesium protect against bone loss and nervous system disorders
- zinc is used against bone loss and to keep skin supple
- natural progesterone such as wild yam cream may be helpful
- royal jelly will help with fatigue, wellbeing and hormonal balance (check for allergy).

Lifestyle factors

- exercise moderately and regularly
- enjoy this time of your life by taking the necessary steps to make this transition as symptom-free as possible

- ❧ deal with or avoid any stress
- ❧ drink about 2 litres of pure water a day
- ❧ smokers may experience menopause earlier than non-smoking women
- ❧ eat simply.

See also Acidosis, Calcium, Magnesium, Oestrogen, Oils, Osteoporosis and Sleep.

MENSTRUATION

Menstrual disorders include amenorrhoea (suppressed, delayed or light periods), dysmenorrhoea (painful periods) and menorrhagia (heavy menstruation). There are various causes for these conditions and good, natural remedies are at hand. In general, raspberry leaf and *Vitex agnus-castus* (chaste tree) are used to regulate the menstrual cycle.

AMENORRHOEA

Women with low body fat seem to be most affected by amenorrhoea, the term applied to suppressed, delayed or very light periods. Other causes are excessive exercise, high stress, travel and a competitive nature. If you feel as though you're about to bleed but the flow doesn't come, then stagnation of the blood is likely. Other symptoms with this type of amenorrhoea are depression and pain in the lower abdomen.

Allow yourself to be a woman—menstruation is natural and a blessing. Each month you are letting go of the last month, starting afresh.

Helpful foods

- ❧ mochi
- ❧ brown rice
- ❧ oats
- ❧ oily fish that has been sustainably caught
- ❧ beetroot.

Foods to avoid

- animal meat and dairy
- cooling fruit and vegetables, especially citrus.

Herbal medicine

- licorice
- mugwort
- ginger
- *Angelica archangelica*
- chamomile
- *Vitex agnus-castus* (chaste tree)
- squaw vine will help bring on your period, or try a hot tea made from dried ginger, turmeric and marjoram—it should do the trick.

See also ENDOMETRIOSIS and LIVER.

DYSMENORRHOEA

A slow or sluggish liver contributes greatly to period pain, so the first thing to do is take the burden off the liver by avoiding foods and substances that cause the problem. As emotions such as anger, frustration and resentment are stored in the liver, it is also important to identify any issues you have and find ways to 'let go' of them.

Helpful foods

- raw honey harmonises the liver, reduces pain and is great if there is associated constipation—take one teaspoon in hot water daily
- dried ginger is also wonderful as a tea
- locally sourced sea vegetables supply iron, iodine and minerals
- calcium, zinc and magnesium are essential nutrients to include
- vitamin B and A and protein are needed for good menstrual cycles
- essential fatty acids from spelt or barley grass

- spirulina
- leafy green vegetables also help reduce blood stagnation
- flaxseed oil and sustainably caught oily fish are extremely beneficial
- evening primrose oil is great for cramps and pain, as it contains magnesium and vitamin E
- oats are great
- asparagus eases menstrual pain
- during menses try to eat warming culinary herbs and spices such as marjoram, caraway, dill, black peppercorns and ginger.

Foods to avoid

- cooling foods such as juices
- too much raw food or fruit, especially citrus
- refined oils
- fats and refined wheat
- conventional red meat and poultry, especially if it is factory-farmed
- junk food
- milk chocolate
- alcohol and tobacco.

Herbal medicine

- *Angelica sinensis*
- paeonia
- corydalis
- ginger
- cramp bark
- dan shen
- dong quai
- *Ginkgo biloba*
- *Vitex agnus-castus* (chaste tree).

Lifestyle factors

- drink pure water, as tap water destroys vitamin E, which keeps blood flowing smoothly
- eventually the oral contraceptive pill will start to cause problems with your cycle, so avoid it
- respect the old wives' tale of not going swimming when you are menstruating, as you need to keep your body warm during this time
- keep your kidneys covered, and avoid any cold and icy drinks, especially during menses
- when the pain is acute, try taking two magnesium tablets, then relax in an Epsom salts bath with some lavender or ginger essential oil and drink a cup of honey and ginger tea.

MENORRHAGIA

Endometriosis, fibroids or polyps are often associated with menorrhagia (heavy menstruation). Iron deficiency is believed to contribute to menorrhagia, as are intrauterine devices, low thyroid function and a deficiency in vitamin A. Liver problems are also associated with menorrhagia, as it seems that blood is not being stored correctly in this vital organ.

Helpful foods

- vitamin A-rich foods
- vitamin K-rich foods for proper blood clotting—alfalfa and kale are great
- locally sourced sea vegetables are especially helpful
- warming foods, such as oats, quinoa, pine nuts, black pepper, dried ginger, cinnamon and black beans
- adzuki beans are an old Japanese folk remedy for heavy or prolonged menstruation
- mochi will help with iron levels—this is available with mugwort added
- clams help with excessive vaginal bleeding.

Foods to avoid

- those that damage your liver—refined oils and fats, rich food, complex meals, animal meat and dairy
- refined sugar
- too much of raw foods or juices.

Herbal medicine

- shepherd's purse decreases blood flow
- *Vitex agnus-castus* (chaste tree) for hormonal balance
- paeonia for ovarian health and as a muscle relaxant
- mugwort is specific here, either as a liquid herb or a tea, or in mochi
- dong quai as a general reproductive tonic
- liver herbs, such as dandelion root or schisandra
- ginger for its warming and anti-inflammatory effect

Supplements

- evening primrose oil will regulate the excessive release of arachidonic acid, believed to be the prime cause of heavy periods
- quercetin—found in green tea and vitamin C with bioflavonoids, or as a separate supplement—also reduces arachidonic acid
- a liquid iron tonic will probably be needed
- vitamin A.

Lifestyle factors

- check for endometriosis, fibroids and low thyroid function
- avoid using intrauterine devices
- be kind to your liver—avoid alcohol, recreational drugs, preservatives, chemicals etc.

See also CONCEIVING NATURALLY, ENDOMETRIOSIS, LIVER, MASTITIS, MENOPAUSE, OESTROGEN and PREMENSTRUAL TENSION.

MILLET

This grain is lovely for a winter breakfast. Cook with soymilk or water over a low heat and serve with stewed fruit or yoghurt. Add honey or rice malt to sweeten if desired. Gluten-free, it is available as a grain, puffed, as flakes or in ready-made cereals. As with all grains and legumes, it is best to soak it overnight.

This is the oldest cultivated variety of cereal in the world. An important basic foodstuff in Africa and central Asia, millet is rich in unsaturated fatty acids and vitamins. It balances overly acid conditions, strengthens the kidneys, reduces bacteria in the mouth, is loaded with amino acids and silicon, helps prevent miscarriage and reduces candida overgrowth. Roasted, it will help with diarrhoea, indigestion and diabetes. It may also ease morning sickness.

See also WHOLEGRAINS.

MISO
Refer to SOY PRODUCTS.

MOCHI
Refer to RICE.

MORNING SICKNESS
Refer to PREGNANCY.

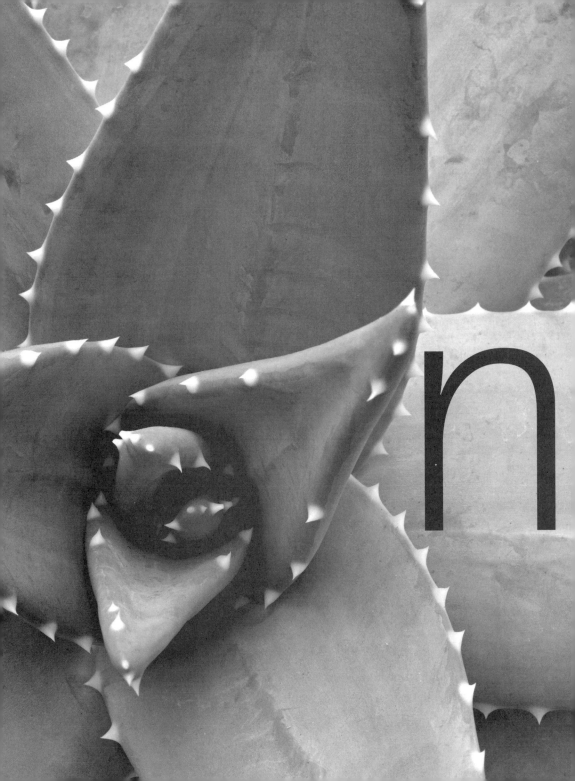

n

NAILS

Your nails are mostly made up of a type of protein called keratin. They are there to protect the sensitive nerves at the tips of your toes and fingers. Your nails should be pink, due to proper blood supply. Any problems are usually indicative of a nutrient deficiency, liver issues or an emotional or physical trauma. The health of your nails reveals a lot about your general health.

Symptom	Problem
White nails	Liver or kidney problems or anaemia
Yellow nails	Liver, respiratory or lymphatic problems, or diabetes (before other symptoms appear)
Dry and brittle	Vitamin A and/or calcium deficiency
Round or dark nail tips	B12 deficiency
Horizontal or vertical ridges	B vitamin deficiency, severe stress or a tendency to develop arthritis
Thick nails	Poor circulation or thyroid disease
Wide, square nails	Hormonal imbalance
Blue moons at base of nail	Lung problems, heavy metal poisoning or rheumatoid arthritis
Splitting	Reduced hydrochloric acid production
Fungus under nail	Candida
White spots	Zinc deficiency
Concave or vertical ridges	Iron deficiency or poor general health
Inflammation around nail bed	Vitamin C deficiency or arthritis
Pitted	Tendency to hair loss or baldness
No moons	Overactive thyroid
Brittle nails	Thyroid problems, iron deficiency or poor circulation
Cut and cracked nails	Dehydration—drink more water

Helpful foods

🥬 those high in protein from sources such as legumes, grains, nuts, seeds and locally sourced sea vegetables

- locally sourced sea vegetables are helpful due to their high content of protein, iodine and minerals
- broccoli, fish and onions are high in silicon and sulfur, which help with nail health
- carrot juice is very high in calcium and phosphorus, which strengthens nails.

Herbal medicine

- silica or horsetail for their high silicon content—needed for strong hair, bones and nails
- calcium and magnesium for nail growth
- iron supplement—liquid is best
- essential fatty acids from flaxseed oil and soy products
- royal jelly (check for allergy), parsley or pumpkin seeds for healthy hair, skin and nails.

Lifestyle factors

- avoid chemicals on your hands, as they dry them out, cause nail problems and may lead to contact dermatitis
- use oil to push back your cuticles—don't cut them, as this is harsh, irritating and may cause an infection
- use a natural hand and nail cream almost daily
- avoid 'buffing' your nails, as it really weakens them
- avoid false nails, which are very damaging to your nails and overall health (just being in the salon is toxic enough)
- use a natural nail polish—there are a few available now, thank goodness; leave the polish off occasionally so your nails can breathe
- cut your nails with clippers, avoiding a nail file, which will weaken your nails; keep them fairly short.

NATTO MISO
Refer to SOY PRODUCTS.

NORI
Refer to SEA VEGETABLES.

NUTRIENTS IN FOOD
Below are good sources of essential nutrients in food.

Calcium	
Almonds, raw	Parsley
Arame	Pinto beans
Broccoli	Quinoa
Chia seeds	Salmon
Chickpeas	Sardines
Dandelion greens	Sesame seeds, unhulled
Figs, sun-dried	Soybeans
Hazelnuts	Sunflower seeds
Kale	Tahini
Kelp	Tofu
Kombu	Wakame
Miso paste	Watercress
Non-fat yoghurt	Wheatgrass and barley grass, dried
Nori	

Fibre	
Apples, dried	Lima beans
Chickpeas	Miso
Figs	Pears, dried
Goji berries	Raw cacao
Kale	Triticale, raw
Kidney beans	
Lentils	

Folic acid (folate)

Adzuki beans	Navy beans
Black beans	Pinto beans
Chickpeas	Rosehips
Leafy green vegetables	Spinach
Lentils	Wheatgerm
Mung beans	

Iron

Alfalfa	Natto miso
Arame	Parsley
Broccoli	Pumpkin seeds
Cherries	Quinoa
Chickpeas	Sea vegetables
Kale	Soybeans
Micro-algae	Tofu

Magnesium

Leafy green vegetables	Sea vegetables
Kale	Sunflower seeds
Natto miso	Tofu
Pumpkin seeds	Wheatgerm
Quinoa	
Raw cacao	
Rice bran	

Protein

Amaranth	Nori sheets
Eggs	Nuts
Fish	Quinoa
Goats milk	Spirulina
Goji berries	Tempeh
Legumes	Tofu

Vitamin A

Beet greens	Spirulina
Carrot juice	Sweet potato
Carrots, raw	Tempeh
Goji berries	Tofu
Mango	Turnip greens
Nori	
Spinach	

Vitamin B12

Chlorella	Nuts
Dried fruit	Seeds
Kombu	Shiitake mushrooms
Leafy green vegetables	Sourdough bread
Molasses	Spirulina
Natto miso	Tempeh
Nori	Tofu
Nutritional yeast	Wakame

Vitamin C

Acerola cherries	Orange juice
Blackcurrants	Red capsicum
Broccoli	Rockmelon
Goji berries	Strawberries
Guava	
Kiwifruit	

Vitamin E

Almond oil	Olive oil
Hazelnut oil	Sunflower oil

Zinc	
Alfalfa	Sardines
Brown rice	Seafood
Legumes	Soybeans
Miso	Squash seeds
Mushrooms	Sunflower seeds
Oysters	Wheatgerm
Pecans	Wholegrains
Pepitas	

See also BABY, NUTRITION; CALCIUM; CHILDREN, NUTRITION; FOLIC ACID; IRON; MAGNESIUM; VITAMINS; and ZINC.

NUTS

Most of us know how good nuts are for us. We know to buy them unsalted, and preferably still in their shell. This retains the integrity of the fatty acids and, unless they are organically grown, somewhat protects them from the pesticides used to grow them.

A small cup full of mixed nuts contains about 3780 kilojoules, and most of these are from fat. Good fat nonetheless, but moderation is still required. A handful (ten) is enough for one serve per day. These good oils are wonderful for your health. So many things will improve—your hair and skin, cardiovascular and reproductive systems, immunity and so much more.

Like all food, unless it is certified organic, nuts are sprayed with toxic chemicals. As most pesticides are hydrophobic, they are absorbed in the lipidic matrix of the nuts (fat content 50–70 per cent) and pass on to you when you consume them.

Almonds High in vitamin E, almonds have more magnesium than most nuts. A quarter of a cup of whole almonds has almost the same amount of calcium as a quarter of a cup of milk. They also contain 14 grams of fat, 6 grams of protein and more than 35 per cent of your recommended daily intake (RDI) of vitamin E.

Brazil nuts These are the best nuts for men because they are high in selenium, which may protect them against prostate cancer. They contain 798 kilojoules, 19 grams of fat and 4 grams of protein. A 28 gram serving of Brazil nuts contains nearly ten times the RDI of selenium.

Cashews Cashews have more magnesium than almonds. Most of the unsaturated fat in cashews is oleic acid, which is the same fat that's in heart-healthy olive oil. With 672 kilojoules, 13 grams of fat and 4 grams of protein, cashews contain more than 5 per cent of the RDI.

Hazelnuts One of the highest sources of vitamin E, hazelnuts contain 748 kilojoules, 17 grams of fat and 4.24 grams of protein.

Macadamia nuts One serve of macadamia nuts contains 6 per cent of the RDI of iron and more than 20 per cent of the RDI of thiamine. They contain 840 kilojoules, 22 grams of fat and 2 grams of protein.

Pecans 'Pecan' is from an Algonquin word, meaning a nut that requires a stone to crack it. Pecans contain 840 kilojoules, 20 grams of fat and 3 grams of protein.

Pine nuts There are more than 140 species of pine trees that produce cones containing edible seeds or nuts. They contain 836 kilojoules, 19 grams of fat and 3.88 grams of protein.

Pistachios Very high in antioxidants and vitamins, the pistachio nut is one of the oldest known edible nuts, dating back at least 9000 years. Pistachios contain 672 kilojoules, 13 grams of fat and 6 grams of protein. Pistachio's antioxidants include lutein and betacarotene.

Walnuts The walnut is the only nut with alpha-linolenic acid, an omega 3 fatty acid. It also has vitamin E and magnesium, 798 kilojoules, 18 grams of fat and 4 grams of protein. Walnuts have special anti-inflammatory benefits because they contain some tannins and quinone, which is found in almost no other food.

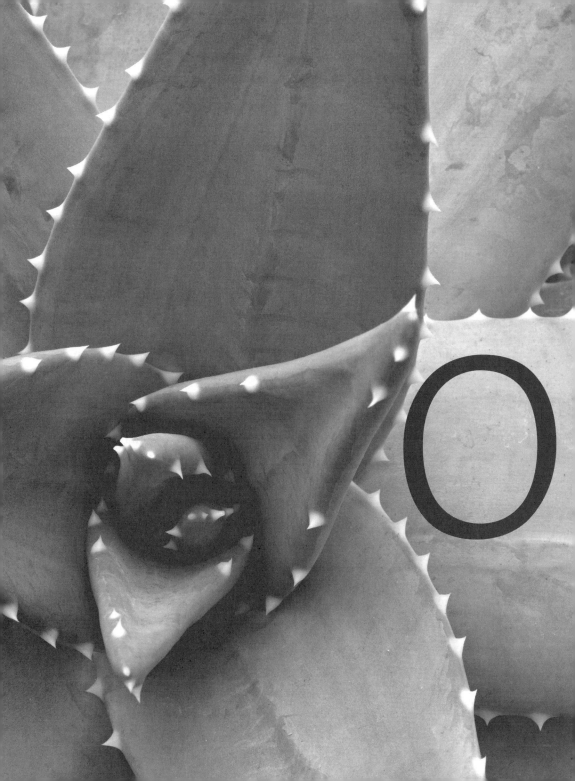

OATS

Oats aid the nervous and reproductive systems, strengthen heart muscles and remove cholesterol from arteries and the gastrointestinal tract. They are helpful for indigestion, sexual dysfunction, abdominal bloating, diabetes, nervous tension and dysentery. They help with bone density and renew connective tissue, and are high in silicon as well. Oats also contain phosphorus, which is required for brain and nerve formation in children. Available as a flour, meal, flakes, milk and bran, oats contain gluten.

See also WHOLEGRAINS.

OESTROGEN

Oestrogen is known as a predominantly female hormone. There are receptor sites in your body that take hold of either the preferable phyto-oestrogens ('phyto', from the Greek, means plant) or the nasty xeno-oestrogens ('xeno', also from the Greek, means 'foreign' or 'stranger'). Your body can't tell the difference between them, which is why it is important to include plenty of phyto-oestrogens so the xeno-oestrogens can't be taken up.

Xeno-oestrogens are found in pollution, synthetic hormones, fertilisers, cleaning and body products, pesticides and growth hormones. If you inhale, ingest or otherwise absorb more xeno- than phyto-oestrogens (sourced from plants), you will experience symptoms of hormonal imbalance. These are numerous but include early puberty or menopause, mood swings, dysfunction with your menstrual cycle and sexuality, and even cancer.

Helpful foods (oestrogenic)

- vegetables—alfalfa, beetroots, cabbages, carrots, corn, french beans, garlic, marrow, parsley, peas, potatoes, pumpkins, red beans, soybeans, soy sprouts, split peas, squash and yams
- fruit—apples, cherries, plums, pomegranates and rhubarb
- cereals—bakers' yeast, barley, oats, rye, wheat and wheatgerm

- seeds, nuts and oils—corn oil, flaxseeds, olive oil, peanuts and sunflower seeds
- herbs—aniseed, fennel, hops, licorice, oregano, red clover and sage.

See also MENOPAUSE.

OILS

There are good oils and not so good oils. The good oils are unsaturated and they are divided into two categories:

- monounsaturated—found in olive oil, canola oil and almond oil
- polyunsaturated—found in soybean, cottonseed, safflower, sesame, sunflower, corn and peanut.

The not so good oils are saturated animal fats—found in milk, yoghurt, butter, cheese and palm oil—and trans-fatty acids. Coconut oil also contains saturated fat but its medium chain fatty acids make it a healthy one.

Canola

Although high in fat, canola is lower in saturated fat than any other oil. Like olive oil, it contains a large amount of monounsaturated fat. These fats lower total cholesterol and raise beneficial HDLs (good fat). Canola oil is one of the few plant sources of heart-healthy omega 3 fatty acids. Canola is usually grown using GM technology, so make sure it's organic.

Chia seed

Among its many virtues, chia seed is a great source of plant-based omega 3 oils. Other nutritional benefits include its level of vitamins A, B, D and E; minerals such as calcium (very high), magnesium, potassium, iron, zinc; fibre and many more. Use it as you would flaxseed oil and keep it raw. Use it in salad dressings, drizzle it over vegetables, or add it to smoothies, yoghurt, tahini dressing or hummus etc.

Coconut

This has a high smoking point so it is suitable for cooking at high temperatures. Coconut oil has a distinct and divine flavour, so lends itself to curries, Asian food and bland food such as tofu and tempeh. It's gorgeous mixed with raw cacao and made into truffles or bliss balls (see the recipe on page 165). Add it to your muesli bars, smoothies and yoghurt. Coconut oil is high in monounsaturated oils, so it is wonderful for reducing cholesterol and keeping the heart healthy and arteries clean. This oil will keep you full longer due to its medium chain fatty acids, which are so helpful in weight loss.

Flaxseed

This oil is our richest source of omega 3 fatty acids, almost twice as much as fish oil. Cold-pressed flaxseed oil is consumed by a growing number of people to increase their intake of the hard-to-find sustainable omega 3 essential fatty acids (linolenic). The body doesn't make linolenic acid but every cell uses it. Life cannot exist without it. It can be used for the treatment of heart disease, diabetes, cancer, arthritis, asthma, PMT, allergies, ADHD, irritable bowel syndrome, diverticulitis, inflammatory conditions, water retention, skin conditions, stress and lack of vitality—take one to three tablespoons each day for maintenance, or two to eight if you are undergoing cancer therapy. Keep it raw.

Olive

Very high in monounsaturated fats—shown to reduce total cholesterol without lowering the HDLs, which keep arteries clear of plaque—olive oil may help to reduce high blood pressure and even glucose levels. It is a good source of vitamin E that helps to strengthen immunity and keep skin supple. Don't let it 'smoke'—once this happens, it becomes rancid and carcinogenic.

Peanut

Western peanut oil is quite bland, whereas Chinese brands have a distinct peanut flavour. The oil has a high smoking point, making it suitable for all high-temperature stove-top cooking. It doesn't contain high amounts of any nutrient really. It is normally used for flavour and its high smoking point. Make it organic, as peanuts contain a toxic compound.

Safflower

Of all the types of oil, safflower has the highest amount of polyunsaturated fat, which prevents destructive, oxidative reactions in the body. It's useful for high-temperature cooking due to its high smoking point, and for whenever you need oil but little flavour.

Sesame

Although high in total fat, sesame oil is mostly unsaturated. This is the type of fat that can help lower serum cholesterol levels. Like other vegetable oils, sesame contains no dietary cholesterol or sodium. Toasted sesame oil has a much stronger flavour, so use this as a garnish.

These beneficial oils contain a combination of the omegas, but each has a higher concentration of omega 3, 6 or 9, as listed below.

Omega 3	Omega 6	Omega 9
Canola	Corn	Avocado
Chia	Safflower	Macadamia
Fish	Sesame	Olive oil
Flaxseed	Soybean	
Pumpkin	Sunflower	
Walnut	Wheatgerm	

Trans-fatty acids

When margarine first hit the shelves, we were told of its health benefits. The health claim was that, as it was low in saturated fats, it had to be better for your heart. This is true, to a point. Saturated fats, in excess, do clog your arteries, leading to arteriosclerosis, elevated cholesterol levels and blood pressure. What they didn't tell us was that the fats used to make margarine and other processed foods were trans-fatty acids (TFAs). Nasty stuff! So nasty in fact that the Institute of Medicine in the United States recently issued a report stating there is no safe RDA (recommended daily allowance) for TFAs.

Butter is far better for your body than margarine. If you are avoiding saturated fat altogether, then the alternative is one of the spreads made from a combination of olive, organic canola, sunflower or safflower oils that contain less than 1 per cent TFAs. Butter, by the way, has none. Or you can make your own by blending organic butter and olive oil together and storing it in the fridge—no TFAs in that mix.

Trans-fatty acids are monounsaturated fatty acids that have been transformed from their natural state by being heated to extreme temperatures. Denaturing the oil makes it carcinogenic. Known as chemical hydrogenation, the process changes monounsaturated fatty acids into trans-fatty acids by blasting them with hydrogen gas. This creates oil that aids manufacturers only because it has an increased shelf life. TFAs can be found in high quantities anywhere you see 'hydrogenated' fats on the packet. That means potato chips, hot chips, sweet and dry biscuits, junk and fast food, cake and pancake mixes etc. It is also the oil used in most takeaway shops, heated to smoking point over and over again. A carcinogen.

Your cells can't distinguish between TFAs and other fats. Moreover, if there are TFAs in your diet, then your cells will use these instead of the good oils. This makes it difficult for the good fats and other essential nutrients to get into the cells, as the TFAs change the cell membranes. As you and your cells now become deprived of energy, you will crave sugar and refined carbohydrates to battle the fatigue created by this situation. These processed and refined carbohydrates will send your blood sugar way up, then way down. The result is hypoglycaemia, then increased risk of diabetes, cardiovascular disease, weight gain and a myriad of other health complaints.

In the United States, the threat of lawsuits has made some of the major snack-food manufacturers take all TFAs out of their products. Thankfully, we are now following this example.

ORGANIC FARMING

The term 'organic' means produce that is grown entirely without the use of synthetic chemicals of any kind. These chemicals include herbicides, fungicides, pesticides, artificial fertilisers, hormones and growth promoters. Biodynamic farming incorporates astral constellations—that is, choosing the most conducive of the moon's phases in which to carry out planting, harvesting etc., as well as organic methods. In addition, organic meat, dairy and eggs are produced from animals fed organic feed and allowed to roam outdoors. Buying organic guarantees food is not GM (genetically modified) and hasn't been irradiated. To ensure your produce is organic, look for a 'certifying body' symbol, from NASAA, BFA or OHGA (these vary from country to country).

Conventional farmers apply chemical fertilisers to the soil to grow their crops, spray with insecticides to protect crops from pests and disease, and use synthetic herbicides to control weed growth. Organic farmers feed and build soil matter with natural fertilisers to grow their crops, use insects and barriers to protect crops from pests and disease, and make use of crop rotation and hand weeding to control weed growth. Organic farmers are not allowed to use raw manure. They must first compost it, or else apply it to the soil long enough in advance of harvest so any pathogenic microbes, such as *E. coli*, are rendered harmless by the many organisms found in the soil of organic farms. Conventional farmers, on the other hand, can apply raw, uncomposted manure far closer to the day of harvest.

Due to strict organic regulations, the animals raised on organic farms also benefit. They are fed their proper diet and raised in an environment that is much less abusive than the way they are raised on conventional 'factory' farms.

Studies have repeatedly shown that chemicals and poisons used in conventional farming have a number of carcinogens (that is, they are cancer-causing). In addition the toxic chemicals all but destroy the nutrients in the produce. The use of chemicals makes conventional farming cheaper and easier than organic methods, but organic foods are great for you and the sustainability of our planet. Everybody wins when we eat organic foods. We will not only become healthier but will also enjoy greatly improved soil health and reduced water pollution.

Organic food is less likely to contain pesticide residues than conventional food—13 per cent of organically produced samples compared with 71 per cent of conventionally produced ones.

Fresh produce you'll want to buy organic— these have the heaviest load of contaminants

Fruit	Vegetables
All tropical and stone fruit	Broccoli
Apples	Capsicum
Grapes	Celery
Pears	Potatoes
Raspberries	Silver beet
Strawberries	

Conventional fruit and vegetables with the lowest amount of contaminants

Fruit	Vegetables
Avocado	Asparagus
Bananas	Avocado
Blueberries	Brussels sprouts
Grapefruit	Cabbage
Kiwifruit	Cauliflower
Mangoes	Eggplant
Papaya	Okra
Pineapples	Onions
Plums	
Radishes	
Watermelons	

Nutrient	Biodynamic % difference	Organic % difference
Betacarotene	+14.0	+00.3
Calcium	+07.4	+30.8
Iron	+33.9	+17.2
Magnesium	+13.2	+24.4
Nitrates	+49.8	+33.9
Phosphorus	+06.6	+12.5
Potassium	+07.9	+14.1
Sodium	+20.3	+19.6
Vitamin C	+47.6	+22.7

Are the levels of elements in food important? A 1988 Surgeon General's report states that nutrition can play a role in the prevention of such diseases as coronary heart disease, stroke, cancer and diabetes. The report, *Nutritional Influences on Illness*, cites studies that found low levels of elements correlate with many health conditions. Examples of these conditions included alcoholism, allergy, cancer, candida, cardiomyopathy, chronic fatigue syndrome, diabetes mellitus, fatigue, headache, hypertension, obesity, premenstrual tension and rheumatoid arthritis, to name just a few. The studies do not directly prove causation but do document correlations. The elements found to reduce symptoms are the same elements found at greater concentrations in organic food.

ORGANS AND ASSOCIATED EMOTIONS

Eat in moderation. Eat food prepared appropriately for the self and the season and enjoy a long and healthy life.

CONFUCIUS

You are far more likely to have a balanced emotional state if your organs are healthy, as your emotions and organs are closely linked. Different organs hold different emotions and it's sometimes difficult to know which came first—the emotion or the disease linked to the particular organ.

Often a predisposition to an organ weakness is genetic, but it's interesting to note that once again the nature–nurture debate is relevant. This means that if you have inherited a weak or burdened liver, for example, and you eat the wrong foods and have negative emotions, chances are you will be resentful and have poor digestion, resulting in, for example, nausea or acne.

It is essential that you learn to *listen* to what your body is trying to tell you. You don't get sick for no apparent reason. By eliminating the foods that make you sick and by introducing those that keep you well, you will be happier and healthier and live longer.

The five major organs—heart, lungs, spleen, kidneys and liver—generate and store essence.

Psychological and emotional states also have a great deal to do with how well you utilise your nutrients. When you are under stress you may not digest and absorb nutrients as efficiently, and you may also need higher amounts of many vitamins and minerals. This is a situation where additional supplements may be necessary.

Heart (and small intestine)

Season Early summer
Emotion Joy and happiness
Flavour Bitter—alfalfa, rocket, rye and lettuce
Effects Tongue, blood vessels and face

If your heart energy is balanced, you will be friendly and open to the world. You won't feel overwhelmed and you will find solutions to problems. Worry, irregular heart beats, wild dreams and insomnia are signs of a heart imbalance, which can lead to a scattered mind, confused thoughts, speech problems, depression, poor memory and circulation, and a very red or pale face. The health of your heart shows in your complexion and manifests as self-awareness.

Helpful foods include mung beans, millet, locally sourced sea vegetables, tofu, blackberries, cucumber, raspberries, red lentils, kidney and adzuki beans. Foods to avoid are fatty foods, alcohol, refined sugar and refined wheat.

Lungs (and large intestine)

Season Autumn
Emotion Grief and sadness

Flavour Pungent—onions, fennel, chives, cloves and coriander
Effects Nose, energy and skin

If you suffer from respiratory or colon problems, chances are there is some unresolved grief, either within you or your genetic line, as grief is the emotion attached to the lungs and colon. Healthy lungs help you maintain your purpose and keep arrangements and commitments. The colon, which is the lung's partner in traditional Chinese medicine, is responsible for how well you 'let go' or 'hold on' in certain situations. Unresolved grief will manifest as bronchitis or asthma, or malfunctions of the colon. It is important to address any underlying feelings of grief or sadness to keep the energy flowing freely through your lungs. If the energy or qi is blocked in your lungs, it is difficult to receive energy, making it harder for you to ward off illness. Your lung energy also affects your voice and sense of smell.

For good lung health eat apples, pears, persimmons, lima beans, spearmint, peppermint, sweet potato, zucchini, carrots, figs, adzuki beans, grapes, olives, sourdough bread, millet and rice, sustainably caught seafood, toasted rye bread, leeks, vinegar, yoghurt, lemons, limes, grapefruit, cabbage and organic fresh nuts. Foods to avoid include cold drinks, melons, salads and raw foods, dried spices, juices, raw onions and chillies. Also avoid quick cooking methods such as stir-frying.

Spleen (and stomach)

Season: Late summer
Emotion: Worry and obsessive thoughts
Flavour: Sweet—honey, rice, cherries, peas and carbohydrates
Effects: Mouth, muscles and lips

If your spleen energy is out of balance, you will feel tired, sluggish and heavy. It will manifest as weight gain, poor digestion, flabbiness, fatigue, nausea, abdominal bloating, blood sugar imbalance and loose stools. You will tend to have a sloppy appearance and will accumulate things.

A healthy spleen shows up in a practical, self-reliant, creative and caring person and can be seen in the flesh and lips. Other manifestations include easy bruising, mucus, cysts and oedema, dizziness, poor memory and concentration, anxiety, worry, an overactive mind and obsessive thoughts, and an inability to express your emotions. You are also likely to feel a numbness.

Celery, rye, asparagus, lettuce, oats, cucumber, kiwifruit, rice, peaches, avocado and peas are good spleen-friendly foods. The ones to watch out for are refined sugar and alcohol. Also avoid over-eating, late-night eating, poor posture and sitting after a large meal—be active.

Kidneys (and bladder)

Season Winter
Emotion Fear and anxiety
Flavour Salty—salt, sea vegetables and crab
Effects Ears, bones and hair

Both the kidney and bladder are very susceptible to the cold. Fear and anxiety, the emotions associated with the kidney, can manifest as a feeling of isolation, alienation, insecurity and a belief that the world is not a safe place. This fear can result in deafness, baldness, arthritis and senility. Longevity is determined by the health of your kidneys. Your kidneys also rule your glands, reproductive system, genitals and bladder.

One way to judge kidney health is through your hair—premature greying, split ends and thin hair are examples of poor kidney health. Deafness and ear problems, such as infections and ringing, can also be linked to the kidneys, as can your libido and reproductive health. Without good kidney energy, you will not be grounded or dependable, and you will tend to move from one issue to the next without getting to the root cause of the problem. You may also feel that life is way too hard and be constantly mentally and physically tired.

Deficient kidney energy may show up as knee problems, lower back pain, teeth and bone marrow disorders and problems with fluid distribution, such as swollen ankles. An ache in the calves or soles of the feet and an inability to control urine or semen is another result of poor kidney health. If you have a child who wets his bed, take a close look at his kidney health—it may be fear manifesting itself.

Good kidney foods include walnuts baked in honey, parsley, sustainably caught trout and salmon, leeks, shallots and black pepper. Avoid adding salt to your food and eating too much salty food, such as pork, processed and packaged foods and, to a lesser extent, crab, sardines, miso, soy sauce (which is okay in winter) or raw or cold food.

Liver (and gallbladder)

Season Spring
Emotion Anger and resentment
Flavour Sour—lemons, pears, plums and mangoes
Effects Eyes, tendons and nails

A stagnant liver, which in many cases is caused by over-eating or -drinking, means your qi (energy) is blocked, which can cause feelings of sluggishness. This leads to anger and frustration and a sense of being held back. At first when the liver qi becomes blocked you can be depressed, mentally rigid, negative or suffer from nervous tension, irritability and frustration. When the qi pushes through the blockage all at once, it shows up as anger—appropriate anger should be let go of once it is expressed. In a physical sense, liver stagnation can cause the sensation of having a lump in the throat or neck or distension in the breasts or abdomen.

If your liver and gallbladder are healthy you will find yourself stress-free, calm and able to make decisions easily.

Lemon juice in warm water in the morning kick starts a sluggish liver, and grapefruit, rye or chamomile will also help. Anger in the liver can cause insomnia. This is the type of insomnia where you can't stop working things over and over in your mind—not even long enough to close your eyes. For good liver health try peppermint tea, celery, cabbage, broccoli, leafy green vegetables, watercress, grapefruit, rye, chamomile, parsnip, wheatgrass, radish and locally sourced sea vegetables. Steer clear of heavy, rich, artificial and fatty foods and avoid alcohol, tobacco and late night meals or over-eating. Chill out.

See also AUTUMN, CARDIOVASCULAR HEALTH, LIVER, MEMORY, SPRING, SUMMER and WINTER.

OSTEOPOROSIS

Women are ten times more likely to develop osteoporosis than men. Osteoporosis causes a loss of calcium from bones, making them brittle and therefore susceptible to fractures. Bone mass in women gradually begins to decline after about 30 years of age. Increased age, menopause and a sedentary lifestyle are common reasons for osteoporosis. The symptoms of this potentially crippling condition include changes in your posture, loss of height, tooth loss and general aches and pains.

Helpful foods

- leafy dark green vegetables such as kale, wheat and barley grass and locally sourced sea vegetables help correct hormonal activity
- those that contain mucopolysaccharides (gooey stuff), such as chia seeds, oats and green mussels, to improve cartilage health
- soy products and wild yam cream, natural sources of progesterone, which have been shown to be very helpful
- those high in calcium and magnesium.

Foods to avoid

- animal meat, as it causes calcium loss through increased urinary flow—it is also very acidic, which is a problem in any disease
- the Nightshade family of vegetables—tomatoes, capsicum, eggplant, potatoes and chillies—as these cause calcium malabsorption
- refined fats and oils
- processed and refined foods
- refined wheat and sugar
- those high in protein, salt and sugar, as they cause your body to excrete calcium—protein should be only 10 to 20 per cent of your diet and predominantly organic and plant-based.

Herbal medicine

- horsetail is very high in silica, which is important for good bone health
- rosehip tea is high in boron (needed for bones) and vitamin C
- gotu kola reduces the pain and cause of 'osteo'
- wild yam for its effect on progesterone
- black cohosh for its use in menopause
- dan shen helps promote the healing of fractures
- celery, which is antirheumatic.

Supplements

- magnesium and calcium are the most important supplements for osteoporosis, as both are major regulators of bone metabolism and needed to pull calcium into the bones
- calcium orotate or citrate
- vitamin D and C for calcium absorption
- silica for strong bones
- flaxseed or chia seed oil is essential—take three tablespoons a day.

Lifestyle factors

- thyroid disease, liver or kidney disease, early menopause (either naturally or after a hysterectomy) or a sedentary lifestyle will increase susceptibility
- coffee, alcohol and drugs cause calcium loss, so avoid
- avoid smoking
- reduce your exposure to aluminium, as it affects calcium metabolism
- fluoride found in tap water and most toothpastes will increase the risk of a hip (or any) fracture due to its detrimental effect on our bones
- exercise is vital, especially weight-bearing exercise such as walking and yoga
- get some sun every day; before 10 a.m. and after 3 p.m. is best.

See also CALCIUM, MAGNESIUM, MENOPAUSE, OESTROGEN, TOXIC METALS and WATER.

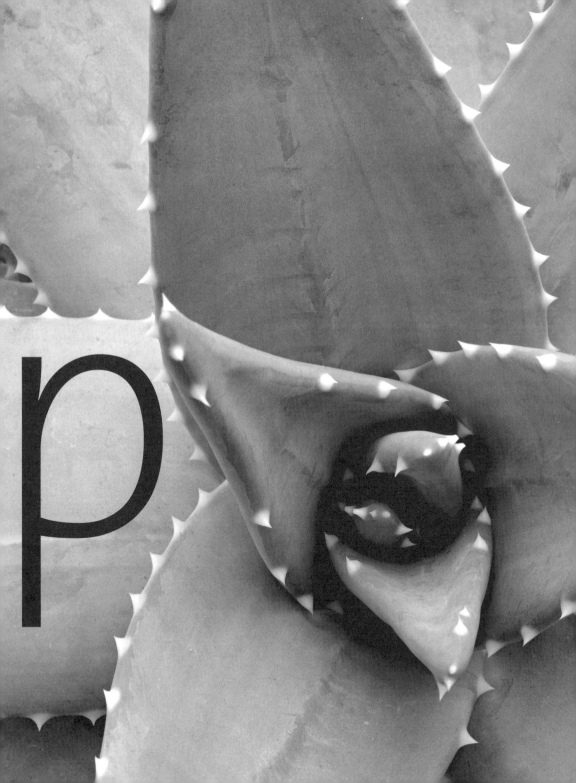

PARASITES

Parasites are more common than you think—the majority of us will be infected, and children are more susceptible to them than adults. They include pinworms (about 1 centimetre long), tapeworms (up to 10 metres long), hookworms and ringworms. These parasites affect the whole body by living off another organism at the expense of the host (us). They thrive in the mucous membranes of the intestinal tract, thereby severely taxing the body and decreasing immunity. They may live in the gut, blood, lymph and/or other tissues.

Ringworms are highly contagious and, along with tapeworms, are the most common. Hookworms enter through the skin, travel in the blood and live in the lungs and small intestines, causing pneumonia, nausea and anaemia. Tapeworms can survive up to 25 years in the body.

The most common ways to get worms is from pets living in the house, undercooked meat and fish, raw vegetables, and walking barefoot in humid climates. Poor personal hygiene and tap water are other common causes. The symptoms of parasite infection are many and, as such, can be confused with other conditions:

- abdominal pain and diarrhoea are common
- gas, bloating, constipation, reflux and irritable bowel syndrome
- malabsorption of nutrients
- food intolerances to fats, gluten (in wheat) and lactose (in dairy)
- hyper- or hypoglycaemia
- insatiable or decreased appetite
- weight gain or loss
- compromised immunity
- allergies
- nervous system disorders, such as nervousness, depression and anxiety, and hyperactivity in children

- pale complexion
- blue or purple specks in the eyes
- white spots on the face, especially around the mouth
- itchy anus, especially at night
- constant nose picking or itchy nose
- cravings for sugar, dried food (especially rice), charcoal or burned food
- eating dirt, seen in children
- anaemia
- decreased growth.

Helpful foods

- anti-parasitic foods, such as beetroot, cabbage, carrots, garlic, leeks, onions, radishes and figs
- a high-fibre diet is essential
- protein-rich foods, such as legumes and beans
- iron-rich foods, such as fish, sesame seeds, pumpkin, parsley and legumes
- umeboshi plums
- onions—they are pungent in flavour and high in sulfur, which helps to remove parasites
- prawns eliminate worms
- lemons are antimicrobial and antiseptic
- squash and their seeds destroy worms
- pumpkin seeds are an old remedy for ridding the body of worms
- sauerkraut is wonderful for maintaining good intestinal health
- pineapples contain an enzyme called bromelain, which destroys worms
- pomegranates expel worms, especially ringworms and tapeworms
- carrots contain oil that destroys pinworms and ringworms
- bitter foods such as alfalfa, rocket and rye are helpful

- the herbs fennel, cloves, sage, garlic, ginger, horseradish, cayenne and thyme
- cucumbers contain erepsis, a digestive enzyme that destroys worms, especially tapeworms
- mochi (pounded rice available from health food stores) with mugwort (a herb).

Foods to avoid

- sugar—worms thrive on it
- meat, especially pork
- junk food
- besides cabbage, avoid raw salad vegetables unless they have been washed in vinegar or citrus seed extract
- raw nuts, especially walnuts
- cooked rice
- refined foods
- dairy, meat and heavy oils.

Herbal medicine

- calendula or witch-hazel for an itchy or irritated anus
- fennel and licorice for colon health
- wormwood, gentian, mugwort, nettles, black walnut and rhubarb root are specific for eliminating worms—NOT to be taken by pregnant or lactating women
- citrus seed extract is a natural antibiotic that inhibits parasites; it may be used for soaking raw fruit and vegetables in order to remove parasites—NOT to be taken by pregnant or lactating women
- herbal teas, such as chrysanthemum, Corsican sea vegetable for children, paw paw seeds and mugwort in the evening before bedtime.

Supplements

- essential fatty acids protect the gut—sources include flaxseed, chia seed, sustainably caught fish, evening primrose or olive oils
- vitamin C for infection and immunity
- acidophilus to balance your gut flora
- colloidal silver.

Home remedies

- soak the pulp of a paw paw in apple cider vinegar for 24 hours, then consume the pulp and vinegar over a week
- soak any raw fruit and vegetables in ½ cup of apple cider vinegar diluted in a sink full of filtered water—this will keep your produce fresh for longer and remove bacteria and parasites
- make a dough out of buckwheat flour and water, roll it into balls and eat it—this will help to eliminate worms
- for ringworms, sesame oil and tea tree applied topically
- eat raw garlic slices between apple slices, or dissolve garlic in miso soup to make it easier for children to take
- skip breakfast and lunch, then when hungry eat a handful of raw rice (after letting it soak in your mouth) followed by half a handful of raw pumpkin seeds and half a handful of raw onion. Wait two hours before eating anything else. Do this for three days, then wait a week and repeat for three days. This is a fairly harsh remedy, so perhaps try the herbal medicine first.

Lifestyle factors

- drink filtered water only
- maintain exceptional personal hygiene
- cook meat, fish and chicken thoroughly—microwaves won't do the job
- avoid swallowing water when swimming in public pools

- wash hands regularly, especially after playing with animals and gardening
- avoid having pets live in the house, or at least on your bed
- have your pets checked regularly for worms—adding garlic to their food will help dispel worms
- avoid over-eating
- chew food thoroughly
- be aware that parasites can be transmitted through sexual contact
- antibiotics create the right environment for parasites, so avoid them
- travel to foreign countries increases your chances of getting worms.

POLYCYSTIC OVARIAN DISEASE (PCOD)

Like other menstrual disorders PCOD is on the rise in premenopausal women. It is estimated that 15 per cent or one in eight women are affected. PCOD occurs when high insulin levels cause the ovaries to produce excessive amounts of testosterone due to an increased production of luteinising hormone by the pituitary gland. The result is a number of follicles rather than one dominant follicle trying to mature at once. Lack of ovulation may result in infertility. When seen on an ultrasound, these cysts look like black dots on an ovary. They are eggs that have failed to properly mature and release from the ovary.

There is also an increased risk of osteoporosis in women who have PCOD, due to decreased amounts of progesterone and ovulation. The increased amounts of testosterone may cause male pattern baldness, facial hair, acne, aggression and excessive amounts of insulin. Symptoms usually present themselves during puberty but may also begin in the early to mid-twenties.

Carrying extra weight makes everything worse, and there is subsequently a greater risk of high cholesterol and blood pressure and seven times the risk of developing adult onset diabetes. Conventional medicinal treatment is the contraceptive pill, which aims at regulating the menstrual cycle. This may cause weight gain and interfere with insulin resistance, and does not address the root of the disease. Naturally and preferably the whole body must be addressed, and diet and lifestyle changes are imperative. Follow the same dietary guidelines as for any menstrual dysfunction.

The symptoms include hirsutism (excessive hair growth on the face, chest, abdomen etc.); hair loss (androgenic alopecia, in a classic 'male baldness' pattern); acne; polycystic ovaries (seen on ultrasound); obesity; infertility or reduced fertility; and irregular or absent menstrual periods.

Herbal medicine

- *Vitex agnus-castus* (chaste tree) will regulate the cycle and decrease androgen levels, which are too high in PCOD
- phyto-oestrogen herbs, such as false unicorn root, black cohosh, dong quai and paeonia, which is specific in treating PCOD as it has a normalising effect on the ovaries
- for related nervous tension, use withania, Siberian ginseng, licorice and motherwort.

Supplements

- essential fatty acids from fish, flaxseed and evening primrose oils
- B vitamins for nervous tension.

Lifestyle

- reduce insulin levels by following a regular exercise regimen and correcting diet
- deal with underlying stress.

See also BLOOD SUGAR; DIABETES, TYPE 2; ENDOMETRIOSIS; MENSTRUATION; and OSTEOPOROSIS.

POTASSIUM
Refer to SALT.

PREGNANCY

This is a time when women need to take extra care of themselves. By the time you are pregnant you should already be in tip-top shape through a good pre-conception care program. But one of the biggest obstacles most women face at this time is morning sickness. It is often considered a normal part of pregnancy, but it's not; it may even be harmful.

Morning sickness is due to the blood being over-acidic, and this will affect your liver, teeth and bones and also create fatigue. Consuming umeboshi plums or vinegar is a good way to prevent morning sickness. Ginger will ease the nausea, as will catnip. Dandelion, peppermint, apples, chamomile, millet and raspberry leaf will also help.

Helpful foods

- cardamom may be used to calm the foetus
- organic chicken and black beans as a blood-building and energy tonic after childbirth
- calcium-rich foods
- essential fatty acids from sustainably caught fish (three times a week), chia seed and flaxseed and oil
- nuts and seeds
- wholegrains and sprouts
- barley or rice malt
- maple syrup, panela (rapadura), raw honey or molasses instead of refined sugar and sugar substitutes
- leafy green vegetables
- celery for high blood pressure

- foods high in iron and folic acid
- vitamin A, found in yellow and red vegetables
- mochi (pounded sweet rice) has been traditionally recommended to pregnant and lactating women for general health
- fibre-rich foods
- kale, which is high in vitamin K and needed for normal blood clotting.

Foods to avoid

- rare or undercooked meat, poultry or fish
- grilled meats—grilling is carcinogenic
- junk food
- coffee
- excessive alcohol consumption
- blue cheese
- aloe vera
- saffron
- pears in excess may cause poor foetal development and miscarriage
- a woman who is pregnant or trying to conceive should avoid figs.

Herbal medicine

- alfalfa, which is high in vitamin K—needed for normal blood clotting
- either raspberry leaf or ladies mantle tea to strengthen and tone the uterus—drink a cup a day
- St John's wort and shepherd's purse will help the uterus contract at birth.

Supplements

- folic acid, ideally consumed from three months prior to conception, to reduce the chance of birth defects such as spina bifida
- iron, as extra is needed during pregnancy

- vitamin C to help iron be absorbed and to ease labour pain
- zinc—a deficiency may be linked to low birth weight
- calcium and magnesium for healthy bones and teeth; these may also prevent hypertension and premature birth
- vitamin B12 builds immunity and promotes growth
- wheat or barley grass.

Lifestyle factors

- avoid smoking
- reduce or eliminate alcohol
- avoid unnecessary medication
- exercise in moderation
- get plenty of rest
- don't dramatically alter your diet
- you will probably experience very strange food cravings—try not to ignore them, as your body knows best.

Essential oils

- spearmint or ginger oil for nausea.

See also FOLIC ACID, NUTRIENTS IN FOOD and UMEBOSHI PRODUCTS.

PREMENSTRUAL TENSION

Symptoms of premenstrual tension (PMT) occur when your hormones are out of balance. This is often caused by dietary factors and/or liver issues. Excessive amounts of prostaglandin PGE2 from too many animal products in your diet may result in your hormones becoming imbalanced. Omega 3 and gamma linolenic acids (GLA)[1] oils control PGE2. Another cause of

---

1   GLA oils (gamma linolenic acids) are synthesised from linoleic acid in a healthy body. Sources of GLA oils are spirulina and evening primrose oil. Linoleic acid sources are nuts, seeds, grains, legumes and most fruit and vegetables.

symptoms is what traditional Chinese medicine (TCM) refers to as liver 'qi' stagnation—the energy (qi) is stuck (stagnant) in the liver. There are many reasons, both emotional and physical, for this. Balanced nutrition along with a medicinal herb called *Vitex agnus-castus* (chaste tree) is essential for overcoming PMT.

Symptoms of PMT are categorised as follows:

A anxiety

B bloating (abdomen and breasts)

C cravings

D depression.

But symptoms can also include lower backache, headaches, insomnia, joint pain, food allergies and water retention—not to mention wild mood swings. Most women experience at least one of the above symptoms, but many experience more or all of them. PMT symptoms usually occur within the seven days preceding menstruation, but can be present up to fourteen days before.

Helpful foods

- those high in omega 3—sustainably caught, deep-sea, cold-water fish such as cod, salmon, mackerel, sardines and anchovies, macadamias, olive oil and avocados
- alpha-linolenic acid also contains omega 3—plant sources are chia seed and flaxseed oil, pumpkin seeds and soy products such as tempeh (fermented soy product), organic tofu and soy milk as well as leafy dark green vegetables
- GLA oils—spirulina, evening primrose oil, walnuts and blackcurrant
- foods high in vitamin E, such as wheatgerm, spinach, sprouts, sunflower seeds, broccoli, cabbage, olive oil and mint—vitamin E keeps the blood 'slippery' and helps with sore breasts, nervous tension, irritability and depression

- vitamin B6, found in leafy green vegetables, reduces water retention and restores deficient oestrogen levels (one cause of PMT)
- vitamin B12, found in shiitake mushrooms and tempeh
- vitamin A, found in leafy dark green vegetables, and yellow fruit and vegetables, such as kale, carrots, sweet potatoes and mangoes
- zinc and magnesium, found in wholegrains, legumes and seeds, and oysters, which are especially high in zinc, as are pumpkin seeds
- good sources of calcium, which include chia seeds, legumes, almonds, broccoli and locally sourced sea vegetables (such as nori) and leafy green vegetables
- vitamin C to help relieve the pain associated with swollen, tender breasts.

Foods to avoid

- those high in PGE2 fatty acids such as animal meat (especially non-organic), dairy, eggs and peanuts
- alcohol, tobacco, coffee, refined sugar and its products
- refined vegetable oils and margarine.

Herbal medicine

- *Vitex agnus-castus* (chaste tree)—dose is 2.5 millilitres first thing in the morning; a 'practitioner-only' liquid or tablet is best.

Lifestyle factors

- check for thyroid imbalance
- exercise regularly
- drink 2 litres of clean water daily
- stabilise blood sugar levels by avoiding refined wheat and sugars—miso, chia seeds and wheatgrass help balance blood sugar

- try to avoid alcohol, tobacco and coffee, especially in the week before menstruation
- check for candida—symptoms include thrush, food intolerance, fatigue and bloating
- be kind to your liver—try to identify sources of anger or resentment, as these are some of the emotions stored in the liver that will contribute greatly to PMT.

See also CANDIDA, CONCEIVING NATURALLY, ENDOMETRIOSIS, OESTROGEN and OILS.

PROSTATE

Prostate problems affect about 50 to 60 per cent of men over 50 years of age. This increases to nearly 90 per cent by the age of 70. These are alarming rates that need to be addressed. The preferable alternative to 'dealing' with this growing problem is, of course, prevention.

Testosterone levels fall after about 50 years of age. These changes cause an excessive conversion of testosterone in the prostate gland. As testosterone decreases, other hormones increase, such as prolactin, FSH, estradiol and the luteinising hormone. The uptake of testosterone in the prostate gland is increased by prolactin. Beer and stress increase prolactin levels.

Prostate trouble can be loosely categorised into three groups—prostatitis, benign prostatic hyperplasia and prostate cancer.

Prostatitis An infection in the prostate gland, due to either a urinary infection or a venereal disease. Symptoms include a deep ache in the pelvis or groin, and/or pain or discomfort when passing urine.

Benign prostatic hyperplasia (BPH) An extremely common condition. Symptoms include incontinence, dribbling, reduced flow, urgency and nocturia (waking to urinate at night). A dramatic decrease in testosterone is likely to be the cause.

Prostate cancer This affects only a small percentage of sufferers. The speed of the onset of symptoms is usually a good marker, along with increasing pain in the pelvis and lower back. Symptoms of prostate cancer may include difficulty urinating, swelling, fever, urinary frequency and urgency, dribbling urine, nocturia and hesitancy with reduced force. To treat it, you need to look at your diet and also supplementation and lifestyle.

Once again, the Japanese diet comes out on top—few men from Japan have prostate trouble. Many studies show that the gut converts the phenolic component of food (including isoflavones) into active hormone-like compounds and 5-alpha-reductase, which converts testosterone in the prostate. Phyto-nutrients inhibit this conversion. The Japanese diet is high in these important nutrients.

Evidence shows that the spread of tumours in the prostate is reduced by melatonin. It is released naturally from the pineal gland at sundown, but only if you actually see it. So having your computer, TV or lights on when day changes into night will prevent this release. Shift work really messes up the release of melatonin, which makes you sleepy. It decreases with age (maybe this is a contributing factor to why we sleep less as we age). Melatonin receives androgen before it turns into testosterone. At this time of a man's life, this needs to be considered. Melatonin supplementation is restricted in Australia to prescription by medical practitioners only. Excessive supplementation of melatonin causes nasty side effects, such as depression, insomnia, irritability and agitation.

Cadmium, which is found in pollution and particularly in cigarette smoke, increases the level of 5-alpha-reductase, an enzyme that converts testosterone to DHT (dihydrotestosterone) in the prostate, causing enlargement. Zinc helps remove cadmium from the body. But zinc uptake (and sometimes intake) is low in men of this age group—this is probably due to increased oestrogen levels, which interfere with its intestinal uptake, and decreased androgen levels. Zinc is vital for proper androgen functioning and has been shown to reduce the size of the prostate. It reduces symptoms of BPH and also inhibits 5-alpha-reductase.

Helpful foods

- those high in zinc, such as pumpkin seeds, oysters, miso, wheatgerm and alfalfa
- fibre found in complex carbohydrates, such as fruit and vegetables, chia seeds and raw cacao powder, goji berries, legumes and whole cereals—it binds to testosterone and eliminates it from the body instead of converting to DHT in the prostate (the problem)
- garlic, onions and cabbage help remove cadmium from the body
- phyto-nutrients, found in organic soy products and plant food, inhibit 5-alpha-reductase (see *Oestrogen*)
- wheatgrass is used for its cooling properties and its ability to cleanse toxins—it is a strong digestive, therefore beneficial for gastrointestinal inflammation
- locally sourced sea vegetables, such as kelp, soften hardened areas in the body and reduce masses
- omega 3 oils such as flaxseed and chia seed will work just as well as fish oils
- those that help combat what traditional Chinese medicine refers to as a 'damp' condition are rye, amaranth, corn, adzuki beans, celery, lettuce, pumpkin, shallots, alfalfa, turnips and raw honey.

Foods to avoid

- alcohol, especially beer, as it increases prolactin levels
- refined or excess salt
- saturated fats
- shellfish

- fried foods
- excessive consumption of raw foods
- high cholesterol can cause prostate tissue to degenerate, so reduce it by replacing saturated fats from animal protein and dairy products with good fats from coconut oil; chia seed and flaxseed oils; sustainably caught, deep-sea, cold-water fish; olive oil; and avocados.

Herbal medicine

- saw palmetto acts as a diuretic, urinary antiseptic and an endocrine agent—it is specific for prostatic hyperplasia, as it tones and strengthens the male reproductive system and is also indicated for all gastro-urinary infections
- hydrangea, a diuretic, is specific here
- buchu is an astringent that also acts as a urinary antiseptic
- couchgrass, another useful diuretic, calms pain and spasms in the urinary tract and also works on the inflammation
- horsetail, an astringent and a strong diuretic, is used to relieve symptoms of the urinary tract, including inflammation, and helps heal the urinary mucosa
- damiana has a testosterone-like action, is stimulating and enhances functions relating to the reproductive system
- panax ginseng regulates hormonal imbalance
- liver herbs aid detox of toxic chemicals.

Supplements

- zinc inhibits 5-alpha-reductase
- essential fatty acids and GLAs (gamma linolenic acids) are essential for proper functioning of androgen pathways
- antioxidants help combat the effects of pesticides
- acidophilus increases testosterone removal through the bowel.

Lifestyle factors

- reduce alcohol intake
- avoid smoking and shift work
- increase exercise
- buy organic produce
- avoid stress
- lower cholesterol levels
- don't eat too many flavours/ingredients together
- avoid late night eating
- avoid over-eating
- retain an active lifestyle into retirement
- avoid pesticides in food, as they exacerbate BPH—another reason to buy organic foods.

See also CANCER.

PROTEIN

Protein is needed for growth and development. It is also used for energy, and to manufacture hormones, antibodies, enzymes and tissues. It helps to keep the acidity in our bodies in check by maintaining a proper acid–alkaline balance.

Amino acids are the building blocks of proteins. Complete proteins contain all of the essential amino acids. These proteins are organic soy, yoghurt, eggs, milk, cheese, poultry, meat and fish. Incomplete proteins contain only some of the essential amino acids. These are grains, legumes and leafy green vegetables. If you combine, for example, beans with brown rice, nuts, seeds or corn you will have a complete protein. All soy products are complete proteins, as is yoghurt.

Good lentils

SERVES 4 AS AN ENTRÉE

2 tablespoons extra virgin olive oil

1 onion, diced

3 cloves garlic, crushed

1 carrot, diced

1 stalk celery, diced

150 grams puy or green lentils, soaked overnight then rinsed and drained

bay leaf

fresh or dried thyme or tarragon

1 litre vegetable stock or filtered water

sea salt and pepper

1 tablespoon lemon juice

½ cup flat parsley, coarsely chopped

1   Heat the oil in a large saucepan and cook onions over a low heat until soft. Then add the garlic, carrot and celery and cook until vegetables are soft. Turn up the heat and add the lentils, bay leaf and thyme and stir until all ingredients are coated in oil.

2   Pour in the water or stock along with the pepper. (Do not add any salt now, as this will prevent the lentils from softening.) Cook over a low heat until lentils are tender, about 30 minutes.

3   Season with salt and pepper, then stir in lemon juice and parsley. Serve with steamed quinoa or brown rice for a complete source of protein. It's nice garnished with a dollop of yoghurt and parsley.

Below are the amounts of protein found in various foods.

In grams per 100 grams			
Fruit	0.2–2	Chicken	15–25
Carrots	1	Red meat	17–20
Eggs	3	Sardines	24
Milk	3	Sunflower seeds	24
Brussels sprouts	5	Lentils	25
Rice	7	Cheese	25
Sourdough bread	10	Tuna	29
Wakame	13	Nori	35
Spelt	15	Soybeans	35
Amaranth	16	Nutritional yeast	50
Quinoa	18	Spirulina	68
Almonds	19		
Tempeh	20		

The average vegetarian/aquatarian (seafood eater) diet easily fulfills the daily protein recommendations set by the World Health Organisation (about 0.8–1.2 grams per kilogram of your body weight). Animal proteins come with the problems of saturated fats, which have been linked to heart disease and cancer. They also contribute more to global warming than any other industry and, if they are not farmed organically, are treated cruelly and with toxic chemicals.

Plant proteins on the other hand are linked to dietary fibre, not fats.

See also NUTRIENTS IN FOOD and ORGANIC FARMING.

PULSES (LEGUMES)

Pulses are an extremely good plant-based source of protein and fibre and one of the top 10 foods recommended for longevity. Cheap and easy to grow, they keep for ages in the pantry. Pulses include kidney, haricot, pinto, navy, lima, butter, adzuki, mung and broad beans, and garden peas, protein peas, chickpeas, black eye peas, soy, peanuts and lentils.

Mainly a mixture of protein and starch with many positive qualities as a food, pulses are low in kilojoules and a good source of complex carbohydrates. They are fairly high in fibre, which helps intestinal action and even aids in reducing cholesterol. Soybeans and peanuts (actually legumes, not nuts) are the most complete protein in the legume and vegetable kingdom. Combining beans with a grain such as millet, quinoa or brown rice in a 1:3 (bean to rice) ratio, will provide a low gas food as complete protein. (See 'Cooking beans' on pages 86–7.)

It is always better to soak pulses overnight to remove any gas and to improve their digestibilty. Beans and pulses are acid-forming foods and your diet should consist of 80 per cent alkaline foods and 20 per cent acidic. All animal produce is acidic, as are grains, so it is difficult to maintain a good ratio. Adding a sea vegetable called kombu to the soaking water helps to alkalise the beans, thus making them easier to digest (sea vegetables are alkaline in nature but at the time of writing kombu is unavailable in Australia, so use wakame or arame instead). While some protein is lost in soaking, the remaining protein is about twice as digestible. Many vitamins—especially vitamin C, B complex and vitamin E—are actually produced.

When cooking the beans, keep the kombu or other sea vegetable you have used. If left to cook long enough, the sea vegetable will all but dissolve. Do not add salt until the beans are soft, otherwise the salt will prevent them from softening.

The protein content of pulses is twice that of cereals (barley, millet, corn, amaranth, quinoa, spelt and brown rice) and almost the same as red meat and poultry. On their own, pulses will lack the amino acid methionine but their lysine content is higher.

Regarding the iron, they contain 8–10 grams per 100 grams and a good amount of B vitamins such as thiamine, riboflavin and nicotinic acid. Potassium, phosphorus, manganese and magnesium are also present.

Unsaturated fats are the major types of fat present in pulses, so you're getting the good guys without the saturated, refined or trans fats.

Whole pulses contain insoluble and soluble fibre. Insoluble fibre guards against constipation, reducing the risk of colon and rectum cancer. Soluble fibre helps to lower blood cholesterol levels, thus reducing the risk of cardiovascular diseases. The starches and carbohydrates in pulses are the complex type, so they are digested and absorbed slowly. This helps to regulate the release of glucose into the blood and is useful for diabetics, who need to control their blood sugar levels. Because of their phyto-oestrogen content, soybeans are believed to have a role in protecting against breast cancer, osteoporosis and menopausal symptoms. They must be GM-free and eaten in moderation only.

See also ACIDOSIS, PROTEIN, SEA VEGETABLES and VITAMINS.

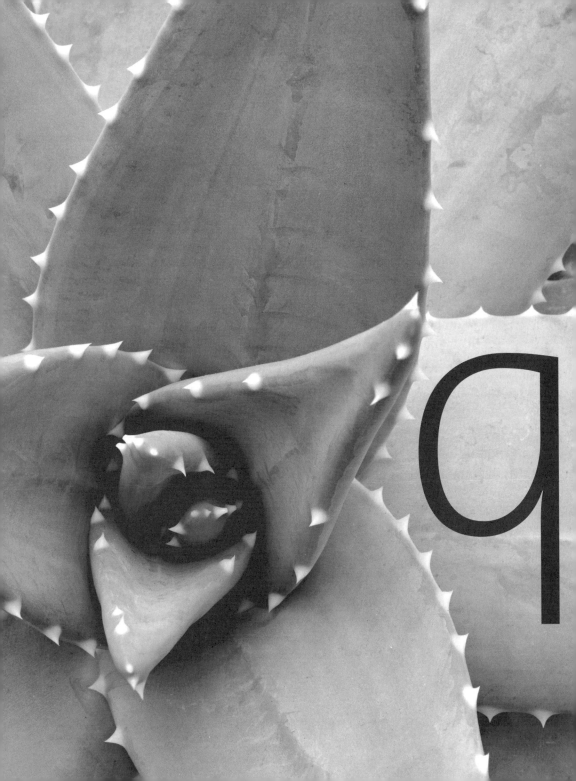

q

QUINOA

The name of this grain, a cousin of amaranth, is pronounced keen-wa, but in South America it's keen-oa. Either way, this is one of the most exciting grains on the market today. Quinoa grows in the Andes at altitudes in excess of 4000 metres. The small seeds are rich in vitamins and nutrients, and were much prized by the Incas, who called quinoa 'mother grain' or 'super grain'. It has only become available to us in the past twenty years, but even so it takes some dedication to find it. Fortunately it is now widely available and becoming more so.

Cook quinoa as you would brown rice, using the absorption method, or cook it with equal quantities of millet, amaranth and brown rice. It can be bitter, so be sure to wash it well.

Quinoa strengthens the whole body and has the highest protein content of any grain (greater than amaranth). It also contains more calcium than milk, is a very good source of iron, phosphorus and the B and E vitamins, and is great for vegetarians. It is quite pricey, so it can be combined with other grains. As quinoa is growing in popularity all the time, the price continues to rise, making it unaffordable for the indigenous people of South America, who have come to depend on it as a staple source of food. Their children are weaned on quinoa milk, and they make all sorts of desserts and drinks with it, much as we do with refined wheat. Please try to source locally grown quinoa. Gluten-free, quinoa is available as red, white or black seeds, flour, flakes, milk and noodles and pasta (be sure they're 100 per cent quinoa).

See also BREAD, CARBOHYDRATES and WHOLEGRAINS.

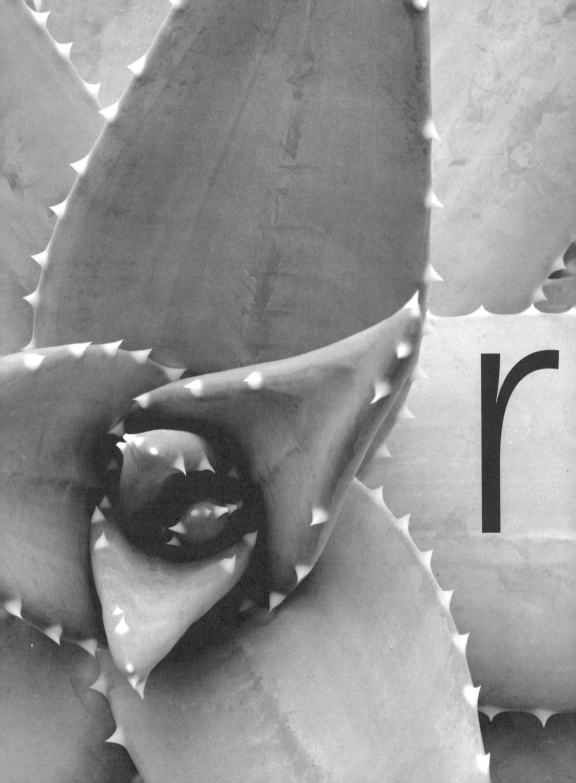

r

RICE

There are so many great reasons to eat rice, which is exactly what most of the world's population does. Gluten-free, rice expels toxins from the body. It is high in vitamin B, so it will help with nervous tension and depression. It replenishes vital energy of the spleen and stomach (thereby improving digestion), and it helps to relieve thirst, nausea, diarrhoea, nervous tension, diabetes and depression.

Avoid white rice, as it lacks bran and the associated fibre and essential nutrients. An old Chinese proverb suggests that brown rice preserves spiritual and physical strength. Try to get your brown rice organic or at least pesticide-free, as it will be much softer than the type you get off the supermarket shelves, which has been sitting there getting dry and old and hard to digest.

Brown rice contains many more nutrients than white rice. To make it easier on your digestive tract, soak it overnight. Below are the various types of rice and their therapeutic properties.

Basmati

Lighter than other rices, basmati is more suitable than normal white rice for those who are overweight or who have candida. Although it's not easy to find, wholegrain basmati is preferable to white basmati, as white lacks nutrients—they have been removed by refinement.

Black glutinous rice

This rice has the bran intact. Under the black coat the grain is white but when it is cooked the whole lot becomes black. Contrary to what the name suggests, it contains no gluten—instead it has a glue-like texture.

Brown or red rice (unpolished rice)

This retains the bran after husking. It has an abundance of B vitamins and is useful in cases of nausea, diarrhoea, depression, thirst and diabetes.

Congee or 'rice water'

Eaten in China for breakfast, congee is made up of rice and water or stock (a 1:5 ratio) mixed into a thin porridge. Millet, spelt and other grains are sometimes used to make congee but rice is the most common. The longer the congee cooks, the more powerful it will become. Cook for at least five hours in an earthenware pot on a very low flame, or in a slow or pressure cooker. It is easy to digest and absorb. It is highly beneficial for the chronically ill, and the strained liquid is great for infants. Whatever is added to the congee—be it a grain, meat, herbs or vegetables—will become easier to assimilate since rice strengthens digestion.

Long grain

This is not as sticky as short grain, so it is better to eat it during the warmer months. Types of long grain rice include basmati and jasmine. Both are fragrant. Basmati lends itself to Indian food, while the lightly perfumed jasmine rice is perfect for Thai dishes.

Mochi

The word 'mochi' means 'flattened cereal' in Japanese. It is a pounded sweet rice product that is widely used in Japan as a medicinal food. Easy to digest, mochi is used for anaemia and enriches the quality and quantity of mother's milk. It also strengthens bladder muscles and is good for bed-wetting children.

Short grain

Recommended for the nervous or frail person, this rice is a better choice in the cooler seasons. Chewier than long grain rice, it also has a nuttier flavour.

Sweet rice

Containing more protein and fat than any other rice, sweet rice also contains gluten, but it is easy to digest. It increases energy, reduces frequent or excessive urination and diarrhoea, and is helpful for diabetics.

Wild rice

Related to corn and not really rice at all, wild rice benefits the kidneys and bladder. Include it in your diet in the cooler months. Wild rice is sometimes mixed with other types of grain.

See also WHOLEGRAINS.

ROYAL JELLY AND BEE POLLEN

Caution: Extreme allergic reactions are possible in some people if they ingest even the smallest of amounts of royal jelly or bee pollen, so test first.

Royal jelly, the sole food of the queen bee, is secreted by young nurse bees between their sixth and twelfth day of life. It is naturally created when pollen and honey are combined, then refined in the glands of the nurse bee. It contains all the B vitamins as well as minerals, enzymes, hormones, 18 of the 22 amino acids, antibacterial and antibiotic components and vitamins A, C, D and E. It has similar applications to that of bee pollen but it also has a strong effect on the glandular and reproductive systems of both sexes.

Bee pollen is a rich source of protein and vitamin B12. It is one of nature's completely nourishing foods and contains almost all the nutrients we need, although not all its properties are known. It may be used effectively for improving endurance and vitality, convalescence, reducing cravings, addictions and infections, building blood levels and overcoming developmental problems in children.

Vegans and many others feel these products—the bees' food—shouldn't be consumed at all. If you decide to use either royal jelly or bee pollen, do so mindfully, as a tremendous amount of time and energy is required to produce these nutritional elixirs.

RYE

To increase strength and endurance, clean out arteries and improve nail, hair and bone health, it's hard to go past rye. It is also useful for treating migraines and increasing tooth enamel. It is suited more to sourdough baking, as it is a very hard grain. A rye product needs to contain 100 per cent rye (or dark rye), otherwise it is likely to contain added refined wheat flour. This is sometimes called 'light rye'. Available as a flour, pumpernickel, sprouted bread and sourdough bread, rye contains gluten.

See also WHOLEGRAINS.

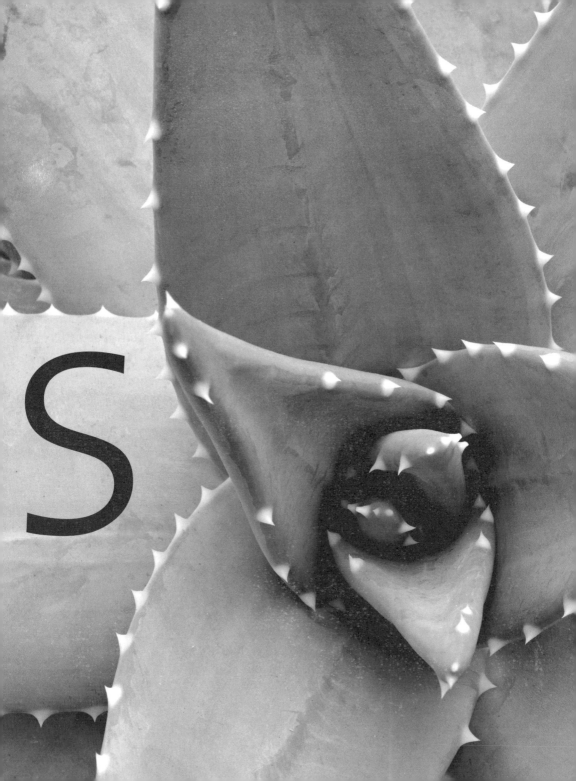

S

SALT

It is widely known that table salt is a contributing factor to poor health. It is also accepted that we consume far too much. What most of us don't know is that a good quality sea salt is actually essential for maintaining good health. The correct ratio of sodium and potassium in our bodies is vital. But it is the pure sea salt we need, not the refined table salt.

There is no place for refined, processed table salt in a healthy diet, just as there is no place for white flour, sugar, pasta or rice. Too much refined salt can lead to heart and kidney problems, PMT, fluid retention and many more diseases and conditions. Maybe we started consuming excessive amounts of refined salt because it was available and also because packaged foods, which we are increasingly consuming, are loaded with processed salt. And perhaps we need to reduce the large quantity of sweet foods we consume. Chinese folklore tells us that an excess of salt promotes greed.

In the processing, salt has been stripped of nearly all its 60 trace elements. Common table salt and salt used in processed and packaged foods is heated to extreme temperatures, and refined salt also has potassium iodine or sodium iodine added (to create iodised salt) and sugar (dextrose) to stabilise the iodine. Anti-caking chemicals are also added so it pours easily. Adding iodine may have started due to an increase in the thyroid dysfunctions of populations living away from the sea (low levels of iodine have been shown to contribute to low thyroid function). Another reason may be due to the fact that as our soils are depleted of minerals, there just isn't enough iodine (and other essential nutrients) left in our soil. Whatever the reasons behind the processing, this salt is detrimental to our health.

Sea salt on the other hand is obtained by drying seawater in the sun. That's it. Good sea salt is grey and available as a powder, crystals or in chunky small rocks. Its mineral profile is similar to our own blood. It has a lovely taste and, most importantly, is naturally occurring. The body easily assimilates its minerals—potassium, calcium and magnesium. Sea salt is used for balancing the effects of excess consumption, including too much refined table salt and animal products, and for balancing mineral stores in the body, and for digestive strength and clarity—it makes your mind clear. It also 'grounds' you energetically.

Sea salt dissolves better when heated, so it is recommended for use in cooking. However, salt is not a condiment that should be served at the table. A good substitute is gomashio, as the sesame seeds in its ingredients help to balance the raw salt. Unlike table salt, gomashio won't cause fluid to be retained in the tissues (leading to high blood pressure and hypertension).

Eating sweet foods will increase your desire for salty foods (think pizza and beer or soft drink, or Japanese food and sake). Cravings for both will decrease with the introduction of unrefined salt. Salt is alkaline, therefore it is craved by those with an overly acidic diet of processed food, animal products, grains, alcohol and toxins. Used correctly, sea salt will aid digestion due to its ability to secrete stomach acids. Modern science also tells us that excess salt depletes calcium and interferes with nutrient absorption, so there is a limit to what you can take in.

Helpful foods

- those that balance sodium and potassium in the body, such as foods high in potassium—leafy green vegetables, legumes, potatoes with their skins left on, millet, bananas (too many will cause phlegm/damp), wholegrains and fruit
- if you've consumed too many salty foods, such as meat or junk foods, try potassium-rich rice syrup, coconut palm sugar, honey figs or yam
- try locally sourced sea vegetables, beetroot, celery, kelp powder and parsley or silver beet as a substitute for sodium-rich foods
- include complex carbohydrates in your diet, such as nuts and seeds, legumes, grains and fruit and vegetables—the sugars break down

gradually, thereby stabilising blood sugar levels and decreasing the desire for salt.

Foods to avoid

- lots of coffee, alcohol and any refined sugar, as they deplete potassium stores
- packaged, junk and processed foods
- highly processed foods, such as white flour, sugar and grains, as the processing of these removes 75 per cent of their potassium.

Lifestyle factors

- salt should enhance, not dominate, the flavour of your food
- cook salty foods such as miso and soy sauces with other foods
- use gomashio instead of table salt
- if physical activity is causing sodium loss through sweat, replace it with juices or herbal teas such as dandelion leaf
- reduce alcohol and other sweet drinks and foods, as these will increase the desire for salt.

See also SESAME SEEDS (for the gomashio recipe) and WINTER.

SEA VEGETABLES

Sea vegetables have been prized, cultivated and used for centuries by many cultures, such as the Chinese, Irish (Irish moss is used in breads, pastries and drinks), British, Icelanders, Canadians (a snack made from dulse), Japanese (who grade the quality of sea vegetables as we do animal products), Native Americans, Hawaiians, Koreans, Russians (fermented beverage and canned sea cabbage), Eskimos and South Africans.

Organic minerals from plant sources are most important, especially if you consume refined sugar, as this devastates the mineral condition of your body. Some of the richest and most complete forms of minerals are found in sea vegetables such as kombu and wakame.

Sea vegetables contain ten to twenty times the mineral content of land plants. Seawater is very similar to the fluid in the womb—consequently, your requirements for proper metabolism are in these little treasures. But many of us in the West shy away from these strange-looking plants, probably because we don't know what to do with them nor how vital they are for longevity. Perhaps we think they may taste like the sea vegetables we see on the beach. Each variety will remove radioactive waste, toxic metals and excess fat from the body. Extremely high in protein, sea vegetables are one of the few good natural sources of fluorine for teeth and bone health. At the time of writing there is much concern about products imported from Japan since the Fukushima disaster. Look for sea vegetables from either New Zealand or Australia.

The following sea vegetables are well worth adding to your diet.

Agar agar

This can be used instead of gelatine to set desserts. It is available in flakes, powder or bars (kantens) and contains no kilojoules, benefits the lungs and liver, reduces inflammation and is mildly laxative. Used to promote digestion and weight loss, reduce haemorrhoids and toxic waste, agar agar is a good source of calcium and iron. It is sometimes referred to as kanten.

Arame

Used to treat thyroid imbalances due to its exceptional content of iodine, arame promotes hair growth as well as prevents its loss. It is also a very good source of calcium and iron, making it helpful for teeth, bones and anaemia. Arame promotes a beautiful, glowing, wrinkle-free skin. It has 100 to 500 times the amount of iodine than shellfish (depending on where it is harvested) and contains more than ten times the amount of calcium than cows milk. Its protein is easy to digest and it is great to eat as a pickle.

Bladderwrack

This is considered the ultimate medicine for low thyroid function. Due to its ability to keep the blood free of clots, it is also wonderful for weight loss and heart problems.

Dulse

Dulse is very high in iodine, and is traditionally used to reduce fevers and sea-sickness. It is helpful where the herpes virus is present and is usually used in soups or as a condiment.

Hijiki

This is a good source of iron, iodine, calcium and vitamins B1 and B3. It is used to eliminate yellow or green phlegm and detoxify the blood, and also for thyroid problems, blood sugar imbalances, weight loss, bone and teeth health, hormonal imbalance and nervous system disorders. Hijiki encourages hair growth and prevents its loss, and promotes a beautiful, glowing, wrinkle-free skin. It contains more than ten times the amount of calcium than cows milk, and its protein (10 to 20 per cent) is easy to digest. (Sadly, at the time of writing, hijiki isn't available in Australia.)

Karengo fronds

A cousin of Japanese nori, karengo fronds are sustainably hand-harvested from the rocky shores of the South Island of New Zealand. They grow in the intertidal area and come to maturity for about two months during winter. (Salt and winter love each other.) The purple colour is characteristic of the Pacific while the Atlantic varieties are greener. During harvest, karengo is rinsed in clean sea water to rid it of debris, then dried by the natural action of the sun and wind. Karengo preserves itself naturally, and nothing is added (if you get a good brand). If it's stored in a cool, dry place away from direct sunlight, its natural goodness will last for many years. Eat it as a snack, add it to steamed or stir-fried vegetables, put it in your wraps, or add it to your grains when you add the water, or toss it in salads.

Kelp

This belongs to the same family as kombu. It should be avoided, however, during pregnancy.

Kombu

Traditionally kombu is used to make hair darker, to increase longevity and intelligence, and to promote a clear mind. It is mixed with tamari (Japanese soy sauce) to improve sexual vigour, another of its many virtues. Kombu softens hard areas of the body, such as an enlarged prostate, and reduces yellow or green phlegm. It balances bodily fluids and keeps blood free-flowing. Kombu is great for any hormonal imbalance such as PMT or menopausal symptoms, and is especially good for thyroid problems. It has so many uses, including the treatment of cardiovascular problems, goitre, arthritis, diabetes, prostate enlargement and ovarian problems. It will soothe the lungs and ease asthmatic symptoms, and is used to boost low iron levels and to treat the discomfort associated with candida. It keeps skin healthy and improves the nutritional component of whatever it is prepared with. It is to be avoided during pregnancy.

It is recommended that you cook legumes with kombu; its alkaline qualities break down the fibre, improving the digestibility of the legumes— kombu will alkalise any dish you add it to. Kombu has four times the iron content of beef and 100 to 500 times more iodine than shellfish (depending on where it is harvested). Its protein is east to digest. At the time of writing it isn't available in Australia.

Nori

Used to reduce yellow or green phlegm and hardened areas in the body, nori, along with wakame, has the highest protein content (48 per cent of dried weight) of sea plants; it is the easiest to digest. It is used for any heart problems such as high blood pressure and cholesterol and also for symptoms of enlarged prostate, such as burning or difficulty urinating, and for warts or cysts. Eating nori with fatty foods will help to process any excess through your liver. Nori will clean the blood, stimulate digestion, and improve appetite and iron levels.

Wakame

Wakame promotes hair growth and prevents its loss, and also promotes a beautiful, glowing, wrinkle-free skin. It also softens hardened areas in the body and will help with fluid metabolism. Japanese women use it after childbirth to purify their blood. Like other sea plants, wakame will help to clear yellow or green phlegm. After hijiki, it has the highest calcium content. Wakame has the strongest taste of all sea vegetables, so don't start with it. Like kombu, it will soften beans, making them more digestible and, also like kombu, it has been traditionally used to darken the hair and help with any heart disease in general. Wakame has four times the iron content of beef and contains more than ten times the amount of calcium in cows milk. Along with nori, it has the highest protein content of sea vegetables (48 per cent of dried weight). It is easy to digest.

SESAME SEEDS

These wonderful little seeds are a fabulous source of calcium. They lubricate the intestines, thereby helping when you are constipated. They strengthen the liver and kidneys, ease a dry cough and help with lower back pain. By soaking them overnight, then lightly pan roasting them until brown, you increase their digestibility.

Gomashio

Goma means 'sesame seeds' while *shio* means 'salt'. The whole art of making good gomashio lies in the grinding process. Use a sesame seed to salt ratio of 15:1.

1   Wash seeds under cold water and let dry on a paper towel.
2   Roast seeds in a heavy-based pan until they start to pop—you should be able to crush a seed between thumb and forefinger. Watch them carefully while they are roasting as they burn easily. Remove seeds from pan and cool.
3   Roast sea salt, stirring continually, until the strong smell of chlorine has gone.
4   If you can, grind the sea salt in a suribachi (a Japanese 'grooved' mortar). Otherwise use a normal mortar and pestle to grind it until fine.
5   Add the sesame seeds to the suribachi and gently crush.

Tips: Don't pound the seeds too much—they should be about half-crushed. Don't stir too fast. Don't crush all the seeds in the suribachi—only about 80 per cent of them. Gomashio shouldn't have a *salty* flavour. Store in a sealed glass jar. Gomashio will keep for up to a week.

Tahini, a paste made from ground up sesame seeds, is extremely high in calcium. The husks of the seeds contain oxalic acid, which prevents calcium being absorbed, so buy it hulled (with the husks off). It's fine to include the unhulled type, but not all the time, every day. Unhulled tahini is beautifully rich, so it has a stronger flavour than the hulled variety.

To make a condiment using sesame seeds, soak about two cups of seeds overnight, pan roast until golden brown, then add one tablespoon of tamari or shoyu (Japanese soy sauces). Let cool, then store in an airtight container. Sprinkle over everything, including porridge, salads, stir-fries, curries—anything you like. Adding sunflower seeds to the pan will give the condiment an extra crunchy, nutty and very yummy flavour. This way you are also getting a good hit of essential fatty acids.

SINUSITIS
Refer to COLDS AND 'FLU, HAYFEVER, IMMUNITY, INFLAMMATORY CONDITIONS and LIVER.

SKINCARE, NATURAL
Your skin is an organ in its own right; in fact, it is the largest organ of your body. There are some specific skin-related disorders but a number of symptoms are a result of internal problems. It is practically impossible to have beautiful, healthy skin if your diet is poor. You need not only a balanced diet but also adequate rest, good skincare using natural products and minimal stress along with regular exercise and a positive outlook. It's little wonder that most of us complain about our skin in today's rush, rush, rush society. Less than beautiful skin may be due to something more chronic or it may be that you've had too much to drink the night before (or the year before), or just missed a good night's sleep.

Age range and characteristics
20s Your skin starts to lose moisture and fine lines begin to appear around the eyes and lips.
30s Collagen and elastin begin to break down and skin pigmentations begin to appear.

40s Deeper lines begin to appear around the eyes and mouth. The skin is not so elastic and it needs added nutrients and attention.

50s plus The skin is less able to retain moisture. Collagen and elastin are no longer formed so the skin looks uneven, saggy and discoloured. Preventing further damage and repair is important.

NATURAL

For a skincare product to call itself natural, it needs to contain only 5 per cent natural ingredients, and this isn't regulated. So the labelling really gives us no indication of how 'natural' the product actually is. A truly pure product contains no synthetic or chemical additives of any kind. These products are very rare. When you do come across an authentic range it will be fully transparent—that is, the company will fully disclose what is in their product. They will state things such as 'vegan, uses recyclable materials for packaging, not tested on animals, organic, no sulphates, parabens, SLSs', etc.

The joy and sense of empowerment you will gain from making your own skincare products is well worth the small amount of effort involved. Your homemade products won't feel at all like the commercially made, mass-produced ones, but you will soon get used to the feel and look of them, and even prefer them. Some of the best ingredients for homemade skincare products are the pure essential oils, which help the skin to function normally and on its own. So if you stop using the oils once the condition is gone, the skin will function properly as long as the internal imbalance has been addressed. Enjoy!

Try the following oils when experimenting with different recipes.

Skin condition	Essential oil
Normal	Rose, lavender, jasmine
Combination	Lavender, ylang ylang, geranium

Skin condition	Essential oil
Sensitive	Lavender, sandalwood, jasmine, rose, blue chamomile
Scarred	Rosehip, lavender, myrrh, blue chamomile, patchouli
Dry	Hypericum, calendula, wheatgerm, jojoba, chia seed, flaxseed, coconut
Dehydrated	Rosewood, palmarosa, sandalwood, lemongrass, coconut
Acne	Tea tree, thyme, lavender, chamomile, clary sage
Oily	Bergamot, cypress, mandarin
Broken capillaries	Blue chamomile, cypress, calendula, geranium
Burns	Lavender, chamomile
Eczema	Lavender, myrrh, sandalwood

Base for your products

Use the above table to make up your own recipes for your skin needs. Use the following bases for particular products.

MOISTURISERS Use either a good quality vitamin E oil or cream, flaxseed, chia seed or walnut, sweet almond oil or avocado oil.

TONER Vinegar, witch-hazel, distilled water or rosewater.

SCRUB Oatmeal, almond meal, rose petals, milk powder or ground rice.

MASK Herbs, leaves, arrowroot, almond meal or yoghurt.

Sea vegetable mask

To heal, soften, hydrate and soothe your skin.

You will need a couple of sheets of nori, a sea vegetable available from Asian food stores and most supermarkets. Cut into pieces and soften by dipping briefly into water. Place the pieces on your face and relax for ten to fifteen minutes. If the sheets start to dry out, you can spray them with water. Then wipe or tone your face.

Honey toner

A healing astringent for oily or problem skin.

Dissolve one teaspoon of raw honey in half a cup of clean, warm water. Next, combine one teaspoon apple cider (or umeboshi) vinegar and three drops of bergamot essential oil, then add this to the honey mixture. This toner can be stored in a sterilised jar in the refrigerator.

Milk and honey scrub

For normal skin, a gentle way to exfoliate.

Mix together one teaspoon each of goats milk powder and almond meal, half a teaspoon of rosewater, two teaspoons of honey and three drops of almond oil.

Lavender moisturiser

A nourishing treatment for sensitive skin.

Mix three tablespoons of sweet almond oil with three tablespoons of lavender water and ten to twelve drops of lavender essential oil. Use as often as you like.

Cream for mature or damaged skin

To avoid using a preservative, make only small amounts at a time.

Mix three tablespoons of vitamin E cream with a combination or all of the following essential oils—evening primrose, rosehip, apricot or carrot. Use daily.

Nourishing night moisturiser for very dry skin

The name says it all.

Combine one tablespoon of avocado oil, one teaspoon of vitamin E oil and ten drops each of sandalwood, rosewood and/or palmarosa essential oils. Apply each night.

Soothing herb mask

A gorgeous infusion of antioxidants and nourishing antibacterials.

Mash or blend about one cup of fresh herbs—such as parsley, mint, coriander and tarragon—with two tablespoons of clean water and two teaspoons of honey. Mix in enough goats milk powder or wheatgerm to form a soft paste. Apply to your throat and neck and leave for ten to twenty minutes. Rinse off with lukewarm water, then moisturise.

SKIN PROBLEMS

It is practically impossible to have beautiful, healthy skin if your diet is poor. You need not only a balanced diet but also adequate rest, enough clean water, an understanding of skincare and a positive outlook. You also need to use natural products, reduce stress and get regular exercise. So it's little wonder that most of us complain about our skin. Less than beautiful skin may be due to something more chronic, or it may be that you've had too much to drink the night before (or the year before), or you've just missed a good night's sleep. There are so many other reasons skin problems occur, but I've tried to narrow it down to the most common reasons and the best solutions.

Helpful foods

- eat a diet consisting mainly of fresh fruit and vegetables, wholegrains and sustainably caught fish
- essential fatty acids from leafy green vegetables, nuts and seeds (especially pumpkin, chia seeds, walnut and flaxseeds)
- avocado, locally sourced sea vegetables and sesame oil.

Foods to avoid

- processed and refined foods, junk food, refined wheat, sugar and dairy products, especially cows milk
- a skin condition is sometimes due to a food intolerance or allergy and the culprits could be milk chocolate, pork, refined wheat, soy, fish, prawns or oysters, eggs, peanuts, milk or other dairy.

Herbal medicine

- yellow dock and burdock will cleanse the blood and help with skin complaints
- echinacea for immunity and blood cleansing
- burdock for liver function, specific to skin complaints, especially boils
- neem for the skin
- pau d'arco for its immune-enhancing and antifungal properties—good also for fungal infections, warts and tinea
- liver herbs such as dandelion root and schisandra, as this organ must be functioning effectively in order to detox waste from your system
- herbs to aid proper gut functioning—chamomile, ginger, licorice and fennel
- golden seal is an antibacterial and liver herb.

Supplements

- vitamin C and arnica for bruising
- fish, flaxseed and chia seed oils are high in essential fatty acids, so they will reduce any inflammation

- zinc for skin health and immunity
- iron, as deficiency increases free-radical formation, thereby making skin conditions worse
- vitamin A (spirulina is great here) for any skin condition, especially psoriasis and acne, and for skin tone
- vitamin D for psoriasis (exposure to sun and sea seem to really improve this condition)
- vitamin E and selenium to improve the health of cell membranes
- vitamin B for skin lesions
- essential fatty acids, such as flaxseed and spirulina for weeping lesions
- aloe vera is good on burns, as is calendula cream.

Lifestyle factors

- exercise regularly
- try to get enough sleep
- protect your skin by always wearing a hat when in the sun
- check for allergies and food sensitivities, and eliminate offenders
- improve digestion
- manage stress—even better, reduce it
- cigarettes, even passive exposure to smoking, have a really drying effect on your skin
- reduce your exposure to the midday sun and wind—try to go out before 10 a.m. and after 3 p.m. only—but as you need some exposure to sun as a good source of vitamin D, don't always use a sunscreen, which should be natural and only used in the heat of the day
- regular alcohol consumption is really damaging to your skin
- acne is associated with poor liver health and dirty blood
- your skin problem may be hormonal; if so, address the balance
- keep your liver functioning efficiently
- drink clean water.

Home remedies

- for scars, apply castor, sesame or rosehip oil topically
- for mosquito bites, use lavender or tea tree oil.

See also DIGESTION, ECZEMA, HIVES, INFLAMMATORY CONDITIONS, LIVER and SEA VEGETABLES.

SLEEP

An estimated 30 per cent of the population suffers from insomnia at some stage in their lives. Lack of uninterrupted sleep creates all sorts of problems. The causes are varied and numerous—low blood sugar may be one, as are arthritic and muscular pain, for example. Obstructive sleep apnoea (OSA)—waking yourself up due to interrupted breathing up to 200 times a night—is the most common reason insomniacs seek help. It affects 10 per cent of middle-aged men and 5 per cent of women, but it is more likely to be about 30 per cent in total. Restless leg syndrome and obesity are other contributing factors, as are insulin resistance, high blood pressure and an overactive mind. Other causes may be:

- anxiety, depression or grief
- stimulants, such as caffeine, alcohol and nicotine
- indigestion
- antidepressants and beta-blockers (heart medications)
- too much mental stimulation
- insulin resistance
- heart-related problems, such as high blood pressure and cholesterol.

Sleep disorders are estimated to cost millions in lost productivity, accidents and health costs, and are usually triggered by an individual's own anxieties and worries. Sleep specialist, Dr David Jankelson at St Vincent's Hospital in Sydney, says that the incidence of insomnia is increasing but professional services are not keeping up with demand. He recommends having a regular waking time and early morning exercise.

Melatonin, a hormone released from the pineal gland at sundown, makes you sleepy. Its production by your body decreases with age—maybe this is a contributing factor to sleeping less as we age. Having your computer, TV or lights on when day changes into night will prevent its release—shift work really messes up your melatonin production. So the idea is to watch the sun set in order to help its production along.

Insufficiencies of the liver will often cause the body to overheat, which in turn causes insomnia, feelings of frustration and aggressive behaviour. To improve your liver health, avoid alcohol, tobacco, coffee, junk food, sugar and animal products.

An insufficient amount of blood being produced in the body can cause insomnia, anaemia, depression and irritability. Include blood-building foods such as leafy green vegetables, pumpkins, beetroots, kidney beans, coconut milk, chestnuts and Chinese red dates in your diet.

According to traditional Chinese medicine, the heart not only regulates the circulation of blood but is also responsible for consciousness, sleep, spirit and memory; the heart is where the mind is seated. When heat rises in your body, you get headaches, bloodshot eyes and insomnia, which can all result in hypertension. If the heart is unbalanced, you won't sleep well. Symptoms include uncontrolled thoughts and irregular heartbeat or worry. (At John Hopkins School of Medicine in the United States, a 2001 study found that sleep disorders may increase the risk of cardiovascular morbidity and mortality.) To control imbalances of the heart, include bitter foods such as grains, vegetables and legumes.

Helpful foods

- lychees nourish the heart and ground the spirit, thereby aiding sleep
- mulberries benefit the kidneys, therefore they are beneficial to those suffering from insomnia
- oysters nourish the liver and blood, helping with insomnia

- pungent herbs—such as dill, fennel, caraway, anise, cumin and coriander—relax the nervous system
- pineapple is useful in summer for insomniacs
- wholewheat, brown rice and oats calm the mind
- mushrooms soothe the spirit and calm the mind
- silicon-rich foods improve calcium and strengthen nerve and heart tissue
- in the evening, eat foods that are high in tryptophan, which induces sleep—these foods are figs, dates, yoghurt, tuna, goats milk and nut butters.

Foods to avoid

- those containing tyramine—milk chocolate, potatoes, cheese, bacon, sugar, sausages, tomatoes and wine—which causes brain stimulation. Especially avoid it close to bedtime.

Herbal medicine

- Californian poppy, passionflower, skullcap or valerian root
- chamomile is a sedative and may be drunk throughout the day—both chamomile and catnip herbal teas are safe for children
- use dill or basil for a calming effect in tea or in cooking.

Supplements

- a calcium or magnesium deficiency may be responsible for waking and not getting back to sleep
- magnesium for restless leg syndrome.

Lifestyle factors

- avoid eating before bedtime
- avoid large evening meals
- exercise regularly and moderately
- reduce alcohol intake

- nicotine is a stimulant, so avoid it
- go to bed when you feel sleepy
- get out of bed if you don't feel sleepy—use your bedroom only for sleep and sex
- don't exercise late at night
- stop thinking by trying to bring your energy/intellect down to your heart—do this by looking down into your chest while your eyes are closed
- avoid sleeping tablets and shift work
- consider learning a meditation technique.

See also CARDIOVASCULAR HEALTH, ENERGY, LIVER, MEMORY and STRESS.

SOY PRODUCTS

First noted in records from about 2800 BCE, soybeans are regarded as the 'beef' of China due to their high protein content. Soy is also an environmentally sound harvest, as 4050 square metres (one acre) of soybeans produces twenty times more useable protein than the land used to raise cattle does. In addition, there are many health benefits to be gained by consuming soy: it strengthens the spleen, pancreas and stomach; cleanses the blood vessels and heart; improves circulation; helps restore pancreatic function (necessary for diabetes); is alkaline; nourishes children (especially through tempeh and milk); and it is slow to be absorbed in the bloodstream, therefore it keeps blood sugar stable.

When prepared and consumed appropriately, the humble soybean provides us with good amounts of useable protein, vitamins A and B complex, folic acid, calcium, magnesium, complex carbohydrates, fibre, essential fatty acids and lecithin. Due to its oestrogen content, it is also beneficial in reducing menopausal symptoms.

Soybeans contain little, if any, saturated fat. The richest natural vegetable food, the soybean is the only pulse that contains protein (20 to 35 per cent), complex carbohydrates, vitamin A, niacin, riboflavin (B group), potassium, calcium, magnesium and iron. Soybeans are among the hardest dried beans, and they need at least fifteen hours' soaking time and a long cooking time before they are edible. They contain a trypsin (digestive enzyme) inhibitor, which may be destroyed through long soaking and cooking, before the protein is available to the body. This may explain why in the Orient they are processed into readily digestible products—tofu and soymilk, which are both unfermented, and fermented products.

Too many unfermented soy products are very difficult to digest, and they leach calcium out of your body, causing all sorts of digestive complaints. These products should be eaten only three to four times a week. When choosing a soymilk, be sure to buy one that uses whole soybeans (not soybean isolates), hasn't been 'enriched', contains no sugar and is, preferably, locally made.

On the other hand, fermented soy products—tempeh, natto miso and miso paste—are very easy for your digestive tract to deal with, so eating them regularly is a good idea. They are packed with essential nutrients, such as protein, calcium and iron, along with a good deal of B vitamins, including B12, which is often hard to get, especially in a vegetarian diet.

Buy only organically grown soy products as, along with corn and canola, the soybean is one of the crops that is now grown using genetically modified (GM) technology.

Miso

A fermented soybean product that is thought to have been used in China for some 2500 years, miso is made with soybeans, mould (koji), salt and a grain. The three basic types are hatcho (soybean), barley (mugi), rice shiro and kome. The colours and flavours vary, but as a general rule, eat the darker ones in winter and the lighter ones in summer. The red varieties may be enjoyed all year round. Those with a high-salt dietary background should be enjoyed sparingly.

Miso is alkaline, high in useable protein (15 to 20 per cent), aids digestion and assimilation, improves gut flora, deals with any stomach complaint, increases resistance to infection and disease, is great for hangovers, neutralises some of the effects of smoking and pollution and, according to tradition, promotes long life and good health. As miso contains live enzymes, it is important to buy it unpasteurised, as heating it will destroy the enzymes. Never boil miso; instead add it just before removing the pot from the heat. Transfer to a glass, wooden or ceramic container for storage, as miso will absorb the toxins from plastic.

Use miso as you would a stock cube—to flavour soups, stir-fries, gravies and sauces. It is nice on toast with tahini and honey.

Natto miso

This fermented soy product is made from cooked whole soybeans, barley, barley malt, ginger, kombu and sea salt with *Bacillus subtilis*. It is rich in protein and fibre and contains very little sodium. Natto miso can be used as a condiment in sauces and stir-fries or as a replacement for miso paste. It may contain vitamin B12.

Sauce

There are two quality types—tamari, which is made from soybeans, water and salt, and shoyu, which is wheat-free. Avoid brands that contain additives and sugar or those that come from Japan.

Soymilk

There are now so many soymilks on the market, most of which are not prepared in the correct way for assimilation and digestion. As soymilk is a fermented soy product, it causes digestive problems unless you consume it sparingly.

Tempeh

A fermented soy product from Indonesia, tempeh is traditionally made from cooked soybeans bound together with a mould (rhizopus). There are up to 30 different varieties. It contains just under 11 per cent protein, and is especially good for the frail, deficient person and also children. High in unsaturated fats and low in saturated fats, tempeh contains a good deal of omega 3 oils. The mould used increases the body's resistance to infection. If produced correctly it will contain vitamin B12. Thinly slice tempeh and marinate in a little soy sauce, then fry it in coconut oil or grill. It's a good substitute for fish, meat or chicken.

Tofu

Making tofu involves soaking, blending and cooking soybeans with a natural solidifier (nigari or lemon juice). This process is necessary for your body to properly digest and absorb its valued nutrients. Low in kilojoules and high in nutrients, tofu lends itself to a variety of recipes. It has quite a bland flavour, but takes on the flavour of other ingredients. The health benefits are similar to other soy products.

There are a number of types. Hard tofu keeps its shape, so it's good in stir-fries, curries or on the barbie. Soft tofu is used as a scramble, as it crumbles, or in cakes. Silken is great used in sauces and to set desserts.

SPELT

This original wheat grain from Persia has been praised as being the best grain for your body. As with kamut, it is unlikely that those with a wheat sensitivity or allergy will react to spelt (check first with a small amount). It contains gluten but it is easily digested. Use spelt as you would regular wheat.

Spelt strengthens the spleen and pancreas and benefits the malnourished person, as it is higher in protein, fibre and fat than most other wheat varieties. Spelt is used to treat digestive disorders and boost immunity. It is believed to be the grain most tolerated by the body. It rarely causes an allergic reaction like modern wheat does, which is probably why it is becoming increasingly available in forms such as pasta, bread, breakfast cereals and crackers etc.

See also WHOLEGRAINS.

SPRING

Spring is the time when your energy moves up and out of your body. The food you choose now should be the lightest of the year, full of young plants, fresh greens, sprouts and cereal grasses. Excess salt from foods such as animal products and, to a lesser extent, soy sauce and miso should be avoided. Too much of this kind of food burdens the liver, resulting in spring fevers, allergies, moodiness and sluggishness. If you listen to your body, you will naturally crave lighter foods such as juices and fruit salads—this is to clear your body of the extra fats, oils and other heavy foods consumed throughout winter to keep you warm. That extra kilo or two should naturally come off.

The organs associated with spring are the liver and gallbladder. Sweet and pungent flavours are recommended at this time of year.

Helpful foods

- small amounts of a concentrated sweetener such as raw honey, agave, coconut palm sugar, panela, rice syrup or maple syrup
- pungent culinary herbs, such as mint, basil, fennel, marjoram, rosemary, caraway, dill and bay leaf
- most of the complex carbohydrates—such as wholegrains, legumes and seeds—have a sweet flavour, which increases with sprouting and chewing
- baby carrots, beetroot and sweet potatoes are also sweet

🌿 raw, young and sprouted foods are ideal now—cleansing and cooling, they are said to encourage rapid movement and outward activity in general.

Foods to avoid

🌿 too much oil, fatty foods, meat, dairy

🌿 those that burden the liver.

Lifestyle factors

🌿 the preparation of food should be simple, as spring represents youth and the raw foods recommended during this season are thought to bring about a sense of renewal

🌿 cook food for a shorter time but at higher temperatures, as in stir-frying and steaming—in this way the food is not thoroughly cooked, especially the inner part, but you still need to cook most of your food to maintain climatic and digestive balance

🌿 sweat as much as possible. Some toxins are eliminated through sweat. Be sure to wash off the sweat, however—if your body reabsorbs it, you will be re-toxing yourself.

See also AUTUMN, LIVER, SUMMER and WINTER.

STRESS

Stress is when the body reacts to a physical, emotional or mental stimulus that upsets your body's natural balance. Physical stress occurs when unresolved emotional stress is prolonged and not addressed and/or dealt with in a positive way.

Helpful foods

🌿 organic fruit and vegetables

🌿 easy-to-digest soups and broths.

Foods to avoid

- those that put stress on the body—processed and refined foods
- animal fats (meat and dairy)
- preservatives
- snack/junk food
- coffee and alcohol.

Herbal medicine

- for insomnia, valerian, skullcap, passionflower, hops and chamomile
- for depression, St John's wort, lemonbalm, damiana, saffron and chamomile
- for anxiety, motherwort, passionflower, hops and chamomile.

Supplements

- magnesium, as it is a muscle relaxant.

Lifestyle factors

- do regular exercise
- get sufficient sleep
- practise deep breathing
- identify sources of stress
- avoid recreational drugs
- consider learning qi gong
- take regular breaks from your routine
- take a flower essence.

SUGAR ALTERNATIVES

Refined sugar, more than anything else, destroys the minerals in your body. Remember, the more salty foods you consume, the stronger your craving for sugary things will be, and that by chewing complex carbohydrates properly you increase their sweet flavour. Try these substitutes, but still eat them in moderation:

- rice or spelt syrup or barley malt
- licorice tea
- molasses
- stevia (a herb 300 times sweeter than sugar—available from health food stores as a liquid, powder or granules)
- real maple syrup
- organic dried fruit or coconut palm sugar or panela (rapadura).

See also BLOOD SUGAR and WEIGHT LOSS.

SUMMER

This is the time of the year when your energy wants to move out of your body. It is about growth and creativity. You will naturally wake up earlier to absorb the sun's healing and nourishing energy. As the heart is the organ associated with summer, it is a time to be joyful, happy and playful. Those with healthy hearts are friendly, open, humble and have clarity of vision. In contrast to winter, when dark foods and clothes are recommended, now is the time to get colourful, both in the foods you eat and the colours you choose to wear.

Helpful foods

- salads
- sprouts, including mung, soy and alfalfa
- fruit, especially apples, watermelon, limes and lemon
- cucumber
- organic tofu
- hot spices—such as fresh ginger, cayenne, horseradish and black pepper—to encourage sweat, thereby cooling you down.

Foods to avoid
- cold substances, such as iced drinks and ice cream—these foods are contracting, holding in sweat, toxins and heat
- heavy foods, as they make you sluggish in summer
- too much meat, nuts and seeds, eggs and grains.

Herbal medicine
- chrysanthemum, mint and chamomile tea
- dan shen for the spirit.

Lifestyle factors
- use shorter cooking methods over a high heat with less salt than in winter
- to some it may seem odd to hear the recommendation to drink hot teas and liquids and take warm showers, but this is to induce sweating, which cools you down
- eat less
- get outside to enjoy the abundance that summer brings.

See also AUTUMN, CALCIUM, CARDIOVASCULAR HEALTH, SPRING and WINTER.

SUSTAINABLY CAUGHT SEAFOOD

We have been very diligent in following the suggestion that we eat three serves of oily fish a week. Now it's time to make conscious and educated decisions about the type of seafood we buy.

There was always something romantic, even nostalgic, about fishing. The Chinese proverb—'Give a man a fish and feed him for a day. Teach a man to fish and feed him for a lifetime'—is especially relevant. The idea of individuals fishing with their own hooks and lines seems honest. Nowadays fishers watch fish from control rooms, use GPS monitors to find their exact location or employ 'fish-attracting devices' (FADs) to decide when to catch entire schools at a time. According to Jonathan Safran Foer's *Eating Animals* (2009), a single vessel can haul in fifty *tons* of sea animals in just a few minutes, making fishers more like factory farmers.

Sadly, 80 per cent of the world's fish stocks are now over-exploited or fished right up to their limit. Over-fishing, destructive fishing gear and poor aquaculture practices have a significant impact on our seas, marine wildlife and habitats. Our oceans are now in a state of global crisis. The choices we make today directly affect the future health of our oceans in the way our fish and shellfish are caught or farmed.

Sustainably caught seafood is fish and shellfish that come to your plate with a minimal impact on fish populations or the wider marine environment. We still have a way to go before we can achieve sustainable fisheries. Every year 'bycatch'—the seafood not directly targeted but incidentally caught, then thrown back dead or dying—kills hundreds of millions of animals, including corals, turtles, dolphins, sharks, seahorses and seabirds.

Gone are the days when we can eat seafood without considering where it came from and how it got into the fish shop or onto your plate. Let's help the oceans replenish. Choose sustainably caught seafood, and reduce your intake. There are plant-based sources of omega 3 oils, such as chia seeds, hemp seed, flaxseed oil and walnuts, which will give us our essential omega 3 oil requirements. Let's give our oceans a rest.

SYNDROME X

Although an estimated one in four people suffer from syndrome X, it is currently not widely recognised by conventional medical practitioners. It seems to have a genetic base with a family history of diabetes mellitus 2 and hypertension. Syndrome X patients have an increased risk of adult onset diabetes and higher than normal levels of insulin and insulin resistance.

High cholesterol may be indicative of syndrome X and patients will often develop high blood pressure as they age. It is very difficult to maintain or lose weight when you have syndrome X but very easy to gain it, even while following the right diet. Herbal medicine and exercise are very effective in treating this complex condition.

Triggers

- increased weight
- sedentary lifestyle
- a diet high in carbohydrates, particularly refined
- increased cortisol production from high stress levels
- pregnancy and menopause
- corticosteroid drugs
- family history of diabetes 1 or 2.

Symptoms

- abdominal obesity
- obesity, but not always
- liver disorders
- high triglycerides, cholesterol and liver enzymes
- hypoglycaemic symptoms
- exhaustion and depression
- upper digestive problems such as burping, indigestion and reflux
- right shoulder blade pain
- liver pain.

Herbal medicine

- liver herbs, such as schisandra, St Mary's thistle, dandelion root and globe artichoke

- nervine tonics and adaptogens, such as Siberian ginseng, Mexican valerian, St John's wort, skullcap and withania
- gut herbs, such as chamomile, gentian, meadowsweet and golden seal, a bitter herb that stimulates gastric acid
- gymnema, to balance blood sugar and reduce weight as well as sugar and carbohydrate cravings
- blue flag, which has been traditionally used to suppress the appetite, thereby aiding weight loss
- heart herbs, such as hawthorne, globe artichoke and motherwort
- adrenal tonics, such as licorice, rehmannia and bupleurum
- circulatory herbs, such as *Ginkgo biloba*, ginger and dan shen
- cardiovascular herbs, such as hawthorn, globe artichoke, motherwort and dan shen.

Supplements

- vitamin E to keep the blood slippery
- essential fatty acids from flaxseed, chia seed, fish or evening primrose oil

Lifestyle factors

- eat six small meals a day, trying always to include quality protein, preferably plant-based
- eat a raw salad every day
- a juice a day is a good idea
- reduce your weight
- daily exercise is absolutely necessary
- avoid alcohol
- caffeine can interfere with insulin, so avoid it
- refined carbohydrates such as bread, pasta and rice must be reduced, if not eliminated; eat other high-carbohydrate foods only sparingly

- avoid bananas and other high-carbohydrate fruits and vegetables
- look after your liver
- be kind to yourself
- keep your blood sugar stable.

See also BLOOD SUGAR; CARBOHYDRATES; CARDIOVASCULAR HEALTH; DIABETES, TYPE 2; LIVER; STRESS; and WEIGHT LOSS.

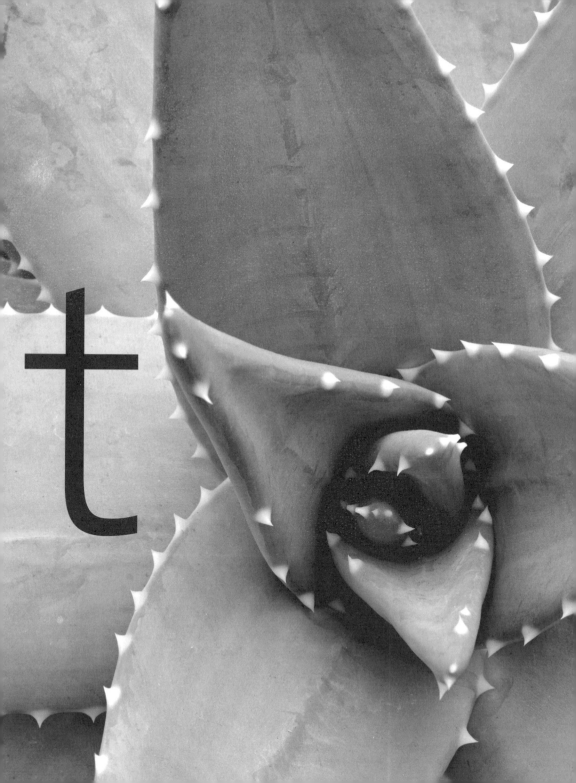

TAHINI

Refer to SESAME SEEDS.

TASTE

Flavour refers to the tastes of food or herbs. Different tastes have different functions, and food or herbs with similar tastes have similar functions or functions in common. The following table analyses the different tastes and their functions.

Taste	Organ	Function	Uses
Pungent	Lungs and colon	Expelling external pathogens	Promoting qi and blood circulation
Sweet	Spleen and stomach	Harmonising the natures of different foods or herbs	External syndromes
Sour	Liver and gall bladder	Astringent	Used for reducing perspiration due to deficiency, i.e. chronic diarrhoea, seminal emissions
Bitter	Heart and small intestine	Clearing heat, drying dampness	Damp/heat conditions. Used for heat syndromes
Salty	Kidney and bladder	Soften and resolving	Used for goitre, constipation nodules and mass
Bland		Promoting diuresis and excreting dampness	Used for oedema, dysuria and oliguria

The need for instant gratification also seems to be applicable to taste buds. Different tastes are detected at different places on your tongue. The taste buds detecting a sweet flavour are situated on the very front tip and the bitter at the very back. One can't help but wonder if our insatiable need for sweet foods is somehow related to the buds' geography, and why most of us cringe at the thought of eating something bitter. A fact to ponder, however, is that your stomach juices are excreted when the bitter taste buds are stimulated. This stimulation sends a message to a part of the brain, called the hypothalamus, to start producing and churning the stomach juices.

Bitter foods prepare your digestive tract to do its work. Sadly, however, most of our bitter foods have had their bitter properties removed through hybridisation. Remember when eggplant used to have dark little seeds? Eggplant was salted overnight then rinsed thoroughly with water to remove the bitterness, but this process is no longer necessary. Most European cultures, however, still value the properties of bitter foods and regularly include rocket, endive, radicchio and fennel in their diets. Another way to stimulate these bitter taste buds is to enjoy an aperitif such as Campari® with fresh blood orange juice or lemon, lime and bitters. The Venetians love an apertif called Aperol®. To stimulate digestion, they usually have it with prosecco before a meal.

> Too many flavours and food groups will exhaust you—your taste buds will have a ball, but your gut will punish you.

TEETH AND GUM PROBLEMS

Periodontal (meaning 'located around the tooth') disease, a prevalent infection in our community, is the most common cause of adult tooth loss. It refers to any problem associated with the gums, teeth or any supporting structure. Diabetes and blood disorders may increase the risk of developing gum disease, and genetic predisposition also plays a large part.

Gingivitis, the inflammation of the gums, is the early stages of periodontal disease. This is caused by plaque sticking to the teeth, causing swelling and infection. As the gums become swollen, they form pockets between the gums and teeth that trap even more plaque. The gums become soft and shiny and have the tendency to bleed easily. Pain is sometimes associated with gingivitis.

Contributing factors to this condition are loose or bad-fitting fillings, gum irritation from false teeth and a diet high in soft foods. Of course poor nutrition needs to be addressed.

Pyorrhoea (periodontitis) develops after gingivitis has been left untreated. The infection starts to erode to the bones supporting the teeth. Abscess, bad breath, bleeding and painful gums result. This is advanced periodontal disease. Contributing factors are a diet high in sugar, long-term illness, smoking, drugs, glandular problems, poor diet, improper brushing, blood disorders, lack of or improper flossing, grinding of teeth, nutritional deficiencies—such as low vitamin C, calcium, folic acid, niacin and bioflavonoid—and/or stress.

Stomatitis is an inflammation of the tissue inside the mouth and cheeks, lips and/or palate. It doesn't usually occur alone—rather it will accompany another disease. In the early stages it will cause swollen gums that bleed, and then may develop into lesions. The two types of stomatitis are also known as oral herpes and canker sores.

Helpful foods
- leafy green vegetables
- barley, alfalfa and cabbage for ulcers
- vitamin A-rich foods—anything yellow, green, orange or red
- vitamin C-rich foods, especially grapefruit and orange
- pomegranates soothe ulcers in the mouth and gums and also strengthen gums

- zinc-rich foods, such as pumpkin seeds, oysters, miso, alfalfa and brown rice
- fluorine from goats milk, parsley, avocado and brown rice
- fresh fruit and wholegrains will exercise the teeth and gums.

Foods to avoid

- acid-forming foods, such as cows milk, red meat, refined wheat and sugar
- too much caffeine and alcohol
- milk chocolate, fizzy drinks, refined salt, fatty fried foods and processed (junk) foods
- black tea.

Herbal medicine

- golden seal reduces inflammation in mucous membranes and destroys bacteria
- alfalfa is high in vitamin K, which is helpful if there is bleeding
- slippery elm soothes mucous membranes
- echinacea and myrrh for reducing inflammation and increasing immunity.

Supplements

- vitamin C with bioflavonoids heals bleeding gums and reduces plaque
- calcium, magnesium and zinc
- vitamin A for healing gum tissue
- vitamin E topically for inflammation and pain
- dentie, made from the calix (top part) of the eggplant, and used to stop bleeding, is very effective for dealing with teeth and gum problems. This is available from health food stores as a powder or toothpaste. It's black, but don't let this put you off. Brush your teeth and gums before bedtime, rinse then rub dentie on the outside of your gums.

Home remedies

- horsetail is high in silica, which helps calcium absorption and increases bone and teeth health—use as a tea for a month
- strawberries strengthen gums and remove tartar—cut in half, rub on teeth and gums, leave for 45 minutes then rinse with warm water
- brush teeth with golden seal for one month
- keep your mouth moist by chewing raw vegetables, breathing through your nose and/or by sipping water and lemon juice to destroy bacteria in mouth and intestines (lemon juice and parsley are also good for alleviating bad breath)
- brush with fine salt if gums are bleeding
- a toothache may be eased by rubbing fresh figs into your gums
- using aluminium-free baking powder instead of toothpaste will neutralise plaque acids and decrease bacteria
- clove oil is antiseptic so it will reduce tooth and gum pain
- aloe vera for inflammation and discomfort—apply directly
- a saltwater mouthwash thoroughly cleanses the mouth—using it warm makes it antiseptic and cleansing.

Lifestyle factors

- avoid smoking
- change toothpaste regularly
- use natural sugar-, fluoride-, artificial sweetner- and sulfate-free toothpaste
- manage stress
- maintain good digestive health
- brush teeth and gums
- floss
- change your brush regularly
- use a very soft brush

🕸 get regular checkups
🕸 avoid mercury amalgams, and consider having any you may have removed
🕸 go to a wholistic dentist.

See also CALCIUM, IMMUNITY and VITAMINS.

TEMPEH
Refer to SOY PRODUCTS.

THYROID
The thyroid gland, located in the neck, in front of the trachea, secretes two hormones—T3 and T4—which regulate your body temperature, thereby determining how fast you burn up kilojoules. Problems with the thyroid gland are related to either under- or over-production of these hormones.

UNDERACTIVE THYROID
This is most commonly caused by a condition called Hashimoto's disease. It is mostly women who suffer from it. Usually the thyroid glands will swell, resulting in a goitre. Diagnosis is made by a blood test to determine levels of the thyroid-stimulating hormone (TSH), produced by the pituitary gland to control the thyroid. Symptoms of an underactive thyroid include weight gain, fatigue, slow heart rate, aversion to cold, fertility issues, muscle weakness, cramps, dry skin, yellow skin and yellow bumps on the eyelids, hair loss, goitre, constipation and depression, irregular menstruation, brittle nails and low sex drive. Your body may also find it hard to convert betacarotene into vitamin A.

Helpful foods
🕸 parsley, apricots
🕸 complex carbohydrates

- omega 3 oils from sustainably caught fish, flaxseed and chia seeds to keep membranes healthy
- locally sourced sea vegetables—such as korengo fronds, dulse, nori, kelp and arame—for their iodine content.

Foods to avoid

- the Brassica family of vegetables may suppress thyroid function further, so avoid eating too much cabbage, cauliflower, broccoli, brussels sprouts and kale, and also moderate your intake of spinach, turnips, peaches, apples, walnuts, almonds and pears
- refined flour and sugar and all processed foods
- processed meats and dairy products.

Herbal medicine

- bladderwrack is specific for underactive thyroid, and other herbs, like those that support the immune system and liver, are needed to support the imbalance.

Supplements

- kelp is very important, as it contains iodine, the basic component of the thyroid hormone
- zinc for immune, thyroid and skin health
- selenium is helpful in the production of thyroid hormones.

Lifestyle factors

- avoid fluorine and chlorine, as these are chemically related to iodine (they will block iodine receptors, as will lithium)—drink only purified water and use natural toothpaste
- if you think you may have low thyroid function, consult your GP, who may refer you to a clinical endocrinologist—surgery may be necessary,

and the drug Thyroxine® or Oroxine® prescribed, especially after surgery
- apart from medication, nutrition needs to be addressed to help with other organ and system damage that may be present
- smoking decreases thyroid function
- avoid coffee, tea and guarana.

OVERACTIVE THYROID

This is called Graves' disease and is not nearly as common as Hashimoto's, but it still affects more women than men. It occurs when the thyroid gland produces too much thyroid hormone, resulting in an overactive metabolic state. This means that everything speeds up. Symptoms include increased perspiration, heart rate and bowel movements; irritability; nervousness; always feeling hot; insomnia; hair and weight loss; nails separating from the nail bed; a goitre and sometimes protruding eyeballs; infertility; and decreased or delayed menstruation. Both Hashimoto's and Graves' diseases are believed to be caused by an abnormal immune response, producing antibodies that attack the thyroid gland.

Helpful foods
- Brassica family—cabbage, broccoli, brussels sprouts, cauliflower and kale—as they suppress thyroid function
- peaches, pears, spinach, radish, apples, almonds, walnuts, soy fibre and turnip for the same reason.

Foods to avoid
- kelp and other sea vegetables, as they contain iodine.

Herbal medicine

- bugleweed is specific for an overactive thyroid and, of course, other herbs are needed to support the individual's imbalance.

Supplements

- omega 3 oils and vitamins C and E help decrease the inflammation associated with this type of disease.

Lifestyle factors

- avoid stimulants such as coffee, tea (all caffeine in fact) and nicotine
- bone loss may result, so keep your magnesium and calcium levels up—a bone density test wouldn't hurt
- malabsorption due to increased digestion may result, so maintaining a good diet is important
- if you have this disease you will most likely be under the care of a clinical endocrinologist
- have your thyroid hormone (T4) checked regularly
- your heart and liver may also be affected, so keep them in good health by maintaining a diet high in fibre, plant protein, complex carbohydrates and leafy green vegetables.

See also IMMUNITY, LIVER and SEA VEGETABLES.

TOFU

Refer to SOY PRODUCTS.

TOXIC METALS

Living in a built-up area often means your chances of exposure to toxic elements in the air, water and food supplies are greater. Your body will be affected some time in your life. Exposure to workplace toxins is a major cause for toxicity, as are environmental pollutants.

Sea vegetables, which have the ability to help rid the body of these nasty metals, are now being cultivated on the shores of Tasmania and New Zealand, making them more accessible. Their ability to prolong life and prevent disease is unmatched.

The most prevalent toxins are aluminium, mercury, cadmium, lead and arsenic. They threaten your health, invade your environment and inhibit your organs from doing their job.

Aluminium

Aluminium is not actually a heavy metal, but in excess it is toxic. Aluminium poisoning can come from cookware, antacids, baking powder, tap water, painkillers, processed foods, anti-inflammatory drugs, deodorant, toothpaste, amalgams, bleached flour, grated cheese, table salt, beer (especially in cans), aluminium-coated containers such as those used for juices and long-life milks, soft drink containers, shampoos and conditioners, and fast food.

Symptoms of poisoning may include Alzheimer's disease, osteoporosis, impaired kidney function and calcium metabolism, digestive problems, nervousness, anaemia, forgetfulness, aching muscles, lowered immunity and reproductive problems. It is recommended you use only stainless steel, glass or cast-iron cookware. Read the labels on products and avoid those containing aluminium (or dihydroxyaluminium). Also avoid foods that aid aluminium absorption—cabbage, cheese, coffee, cucumbers, green and black tea, radishes, tomatoes and turnips—but include sea vegetables, such as locally grown spirulina, karengo fronds, dulse or kelp.

Arsenic

Arsenic is found in pesticides, laundry aids, table salt, beer, smog, cigarette smoke and tap water. Poisoning leads to headaches, confusion, drowsiness, vomiting, diarrhoea, muscle cramps, fatigue, dermatitis, hair loss, gut pain and convulsions. Take selenium, apple pectin and vitamin C, and eat sulfur-rich foods such as eggs, onions, beans, legumes and garlic to help rid the body of arsenic.

Overall, the common culprits in toxic metal poisoning are:

- shellfish—clams, mussels, oysters, crab and prawns (it is best to obtain these from waters near large, clean land areas)
- vacuum cleaner bags, so change them regularly
- cleaning products—try to use non-toxic ones
- insect repellents and bombs
- cigarette smoke
- carpets, which have been known to cause a lot of problems
- pesticide, fungicide and herbicide products—to avoid, buy organic
- tap water
- aluminium cookware.

Traditionally used to neutralise toxins are adzuki beans, black beans, millet, mung beans, organic tofu, figs, radishes, turnips, and salt and vinegar (although these should be taken with care, as they are very strong substances). Garlic, onions, locally sourced sea vegetables, miso, wheat or barley grass, spirulina and apples are also helpful.

See also Sea vegetables.

Cadmium

The sources of cadmium are air pollution, cigarettes, cigar or pipe smoke, plastics, tap water, fertilisers, pesticides, fungicides, air pollution, processed grains, coffee, tea and soft drinks. Cadmium can result in lowered immunity, reproductive problems, low zinc levels, high blood pressure, decreased sense of smell, sore joints, hair loss, dry and scaly skin, poor appetite, kidney disease, liver damage, emphysema and cancer. Alfalfa helps remove cadmium from the body. Also eat a diet high in fibre and apple pectin, locally sourced sea vegetables and vitamins C and A.

Lead

Rainwater, lead-based paints, ceramic glazes, leaded petrol, tobacco, liver, water from lead piping, lead-contaminated dirt, food sold in lead-soldered cans, insecticides, porcelain sinks and bathtubs, and foil wrappers around the corks of wine bottles are all culprits in lead poisoning. This can lead to lowered immunity, reproductive problems, kidney, liver, heart and nervous system damage, gastrointestinal colic, gout, insomnia, confusion, vertigo, learning disabilities, blue gums, muscle weakness, anxiety, poor appetite, arthritis and a metallic taste in the mouth. In more severe cases it can cause infertility and impotence. If you are affected, a diet high in calcium is recommended.

Apple pectin, garlic, vitamin C, zinc, selenium, alfalfa, fibre-rich foods and sulfur-rich foods such as legumes, beans, eggs and garlic are also helpful. Drink filtered water only and avoid smoking, including passive smoking.

Mercury

This is found in amalgam tooth fillings (now banned in Canada and many European countries), fungicides, pesticides, soil, water, large fish (due to chlorine bleaches leaking into our waters), fabric softeners, inks, cosmetics, plastics, old hats, solvents and polishes. Before making the decision to have mercury amalgams removed, have them checked by an experienced wholistic dentist, as removal may result in poisoning. The symptoms of poisoning are lowered immunity, reproductive problems, arthritis, depression, dermatitis, dizziness, hair loss, insomnia, memory loss, gum disease, fatigue, muscle weakness, depression, hyperactivity, mood changes, irritability, excessive saliva, menstrual problems and miscarriage. More seriously, it can cause blindness and paralysis. Think of Lewis Carroll's Mad Hatter—mercury was once used in millinery.

Alfalfa helps to rid the body of toxins. Sulfur-rich foods such as eggs, garlic, beans, legumes and onions, as well as locally sourced sea vegetables and fibre, such as oat bran and apple pectin, should also be helpful. Good supplements include selenium, vitamin E, apple pectin, garlic, vitamin A and vitamin C.

You can eat large fish in moderation since, if there is mercury present, it will be primarily stored in the fat. Grilling first then draining the juices will rid it of any mercury. Avoid tuna, however.

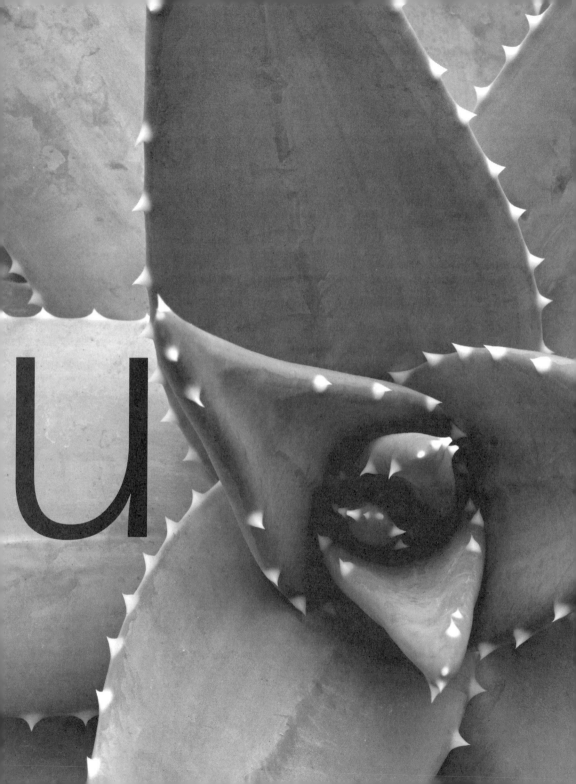

u

UMEBOSHI PRODUCTS

One of my favourite things, umeboshi plums are salty and sour plums. Highly alkaline and antibiotic, they ease digestive complaints, including diarrhoea, dysentery and indigestion, stroke, food poisoning, constipation, too much or too little stomach acid, motion sickness and headache; they can also neutralise sugar, alcohol and toxins due to the balanced yin/yang combination. They also help to remove worms from your body and have a very positive effect on the liver.

In the early 1950s, a Japanese doctor named Dr Kyo Sato isolated an extract in umeboshi that was antibiotic. Just 9 grams could destroy dysentery staphylococcus germs. In 1968, a component of the umeboshi plum that could treat tuberculosis was isolated. As penicillin and other antibiotics were already in wide use, his discovery went largely unnoticed.

Two other umeboshi products are umeboshi vinegar (the brine from the umeboshi) and umeboshi paste, which is used for pickling or as a condiment. Shiso leaves from the beefsteak plant are added. The colour and flavour from these leaves are released easily, since the leaves have been bruised and rolled. Much of the umeboshi flavour and colour comes from these leaves. They are left to marinate for at least six months and up to six years. These types of umeboshi products are precious, as eating just one can stop diarrhoea.

The king of alkaline foods, umeboshi plums contain an abundance of citric acid, making absorption in the small intestine easy. Citric acid breaks down lactic acid (bad stuff) in our blood and tissues. Try to source locally grown products, or at least don't buy umeboshi products from Japan.

Therapeutic effects

- prevention of fatigue—fatigue is usually caused by a build-up of acid in your body which your metabolism can't break down fast enough. The accumulation of acid is caused by eating too much refined flour, dairy and animal meats, as well as by a sedentary lifestyle, as this causes a lack of oxygen in the body. Too much acid makes you more susceptible to diseases of the liver, diseases associated with ageing and infections; umeboshi breaks down acids

- prevention of ageing—umeboshi has an antioxidant effect on the blood
- detoxification—umeboshi supports the metabolism, helping the kidneys and the liver perform properly to rid the body of toxins
- lack of appetite—it will stimulate the normal secretion of your digestive juices
- constipation—take one umeboshi in some bancha tea on rising
- bad breath—has an anti-putrefying effect
- will kill various bacilli such as cholera (after five minutes), typhoid (after ten minutes) and dysentery (after one hour)
- morning sickness—a sign that the blood is too acidic, so take an umeboshi at every meal or use the paste
- colds and 'flu—take one with hot water, and why not add some fresh ginger
- motion sickness—an old folk tale suggests that motion sickness can be prevented by attaching an umeboshi to your navel
- hangover—one of the best ways to relieve the symptoms
- food poisoning—in this case, have an umeboshi with some bancha tea, but if it causes vomiting in order to eliminate the poison from your body, have another cup.

Home remedies

- have as a tea with bancha (twig tea from the green tea plant)
- eat in a rice ball wrapped with nori
- eat one whole plum each day as a general preventative
- use umeboshi vinegar instead of balsamic or white vinegar in your dressings
- mix the paste into sauces or use it as a condiment.

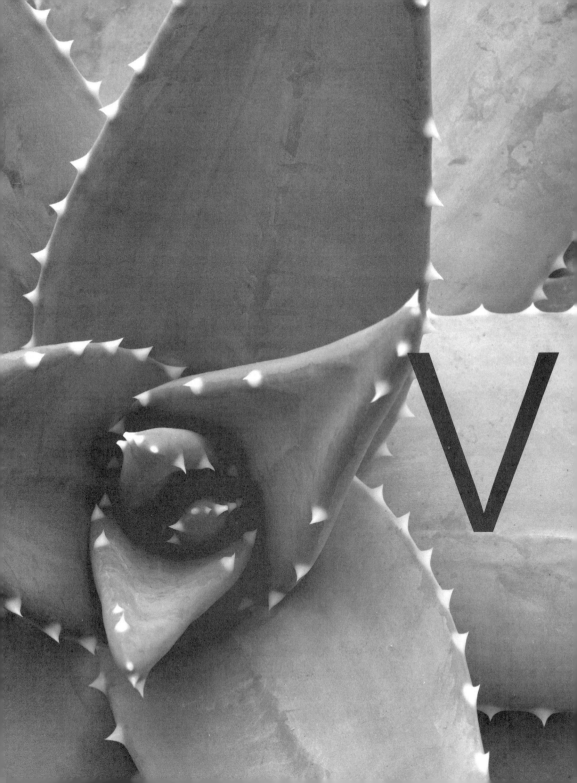

V

VITAMINS

Vitamin A

This is also known as betacarotene, which is converted in your body into vitamin A or retinol.

Sources Spirulina, kale, goji berries, cod liver oil and egg yolks. Betacarotene is found in yellow, orange and red fruit such as apricots, cherries, mango, paw paw, peaches, rockmelon and watermelon, and vegetables such as carrots, pumpkin, red cabbage, sweet potato, winter squash and yams. It is also abundant in leafy green vegetables such as asparagus, broccoli, brussels sprouts, lettuce, nori and spinach.

Uses For eyesight, teeth, bone growth, tissue repair, skin health, as an antioxidant, cancer therapy and to fight infection.

Requirements 5000 IUs per day.

Increased need When pregnant and lactating, with an infection or illness, if a smoker or regular alcohol drinker, and when under stress.

Vitamin B (thiamine or thiamin)

The B vitamins are produced by your intestinal flora, so it is important to keep them healthy. They are destroyed by cooking, sugar, coffee, tannin (from black tea), nicotine and alcohol use.

Sources Wheatgerm and bran, brown rice and other wholegrains, oats and millet, legumes, seeds and peanuts, avocado, oily fish, nori, shellfish, sunflower seeds and leafy dark green vegetables.

Uses For fatigue, irritability, depression and other disorders of the nervous system, to increase intestinal tone, for constipation, mental illness, alcoholism, beri beri and heart function.

Requirements 1.2 milligrams a day.

Increased need Pregnancy or lactation; infancy; high stress; smoking; caffeine, tea or tobacco use; those on the contraceptive pill.

Vitamin B12 (cobalamin)

The human body needs only tiny amounts of B12 and conserves it when supplies are scarce. Vitamin B12 can be stored in the liver for three to six years, which means a deficiency may be present before symptoms appear. Bacteria in the small intestine called 'intrinsic factor' produce it, but this production decreases as you age.

Sources Mostly from organ meats, so thankfully it is produced by bacteria in your intestines. Also found in trout, herring, mackerel, crab, oysters, egg yolk and yoghurt. Good vegetarian sources are miso, tempeh, shiitake mushrooms, natto miso, sourdough bread and locally sourced sea vegetables.

Uses Needed for the entire nervous system, including nerve tissue metabolism. It stimulates assimilation of protein, fats and carbohydrates. Used also to increase energy and stimulate growth and appetite in children.

Requirements 3–4 micrograms per day, but 10–20 micrograms is also safe.

Increased need Age, stress, digestive problems and pregnancy. Weak arms and legs along with mood changes are a sign of deficiency, but usually only in vegetarians. If a meat eater is found to be deficient, it is likely there is an absorption problem.

Vitamin C

Vitamin C is non-toxic, but if you take too much all at once you are likely to experience diarrhoea. This is referred to as the 'bowel tolerance test'. It is a sure way to find out your individual requirements but it is uncomfortable. Vitamin C is destroyed by cooking, oxidation, light, heat and baking soda. It is lost in cooking water, so steam or stir-fry your food.

Sources Fruit (rosehips, acerola cherries, chia seeds, citrus fruits, paw paw, rockmelon and strawberries), vegetables (green then red capsicum, broccoli, brussels sprouts, leafy dark green vegetables, sauerkraut and parsley), sprouted grains, seeds and beans.

Uses For formation of collagen—required for skin, ligaments, bones, teeth, cartilage and capillary walls; for wound healing and to keep blood vessels happy; for adrenal function—helps to produce 'happy' chemicals such as dopamine and epinephrine; for thyroid health and cholesterol metabolism. It is an antioxidant and protects vitamins A, E and some of the Bs. It is also helpful against viral (colds and 'flu), bacterial and fungal diseases, allergies (reduces histamine), asthma, fatigue, slow metabolism, ageing and varicose veins, and improves immunity and sperm motility.

Requirements Sixty milligrams per day, but realistically more like 2–4 grams a day. Start slowly on about 500 milligrams a day, then slowly increase to at least 1 gram, preferably 2 grams. Some people can take up to 10 grams a day. It is used by the body in a few hours, so it is recommended that supplements be split up and taken two to three times a day rather than once.

Increased need High stress, smoking, regular alcohol intake, diabetes, the elderly, allergies, fever, virus, antibiotics, exposure to pollution and heavy metals, analgesics, cortisone, aspirin, HRT, the contraceptive pill, compromised immunity, asthma.

Vitamin D (calciferol)

Sources Cod liver oil, egg yolks, oily fish, mushrooms and leafy dark green vegetables. Sunlight is your best option if you are avoiding animal products.

Uses Regulates calcium metabolism, important for parathyroid gland and nervous system, healthy bones and teeth, and proper heart function.

Requirements The recommended daily allowance is 400 IUs—usually there is no need for supplementation, as you get enough from your food and sunlight.

Increased need Menopausal women, children and during pregnancy.

Vitamin E (tocopherol)

The word 'tocopherol' comes from the Greek words meaning 'offspring' and 'to bear', literally 'to bear children'. Vitamin E is destroyed by heating, processing, storage, freezing and oxidation.

Sources Wheatgerm oil is the best source, followed by other nut and seed oils.

Uses Antioxidant, fertility, circulation, skin lesions, burns, ulcers, varicose veins, anti-ageing, keeps blood smooth and clot-free, improves immunity, wound healing.

Requirements RDA varies depending on body size and diet—somewhere between 50 and 100 IUs is recommended. Don't take it with an iron supplement, as this may destroy the vitamin E.

Increased need Women on HRT, exposure to air pollution, those on a diet of refined and processed oils and foods.

Vitamin K

This vitamin is destroyed by antibiotic use, air pollution, aspirin, freezing foods, radiation and oxidising agents.

Sources Alfalfa, leafy dark green vegetables, kelp, yoghurt, egg yolk and cod liver oil. The best source is your own intestinal flora, so keeping your gut flora healthy is important.

Uses For normal blood clotting, heavy menstruation, period pain; newborns are currently injected with vitamin K to prevent haemorrhage; for morning sickness; to control fermentation of food, so it is sometimes used as a preservative.

Requirements Supplementation is not recommended and there is no official RDA—we seem to get enough from food. It's contraindicated if you're on blood-thinning medication.

Vitamin U

Little is known about this vitamin, even today.

Sources Raw cabbage and maybe comfrey root.

Uses For the healing of ulcers in the intestinal tract and skin, and by lactating women suffering with mastitis (with great results—steam whole cabbage leaves, let cool, then place over affected breast).

Requirements Not known.

See also NUTRIENTS IN FOODS.

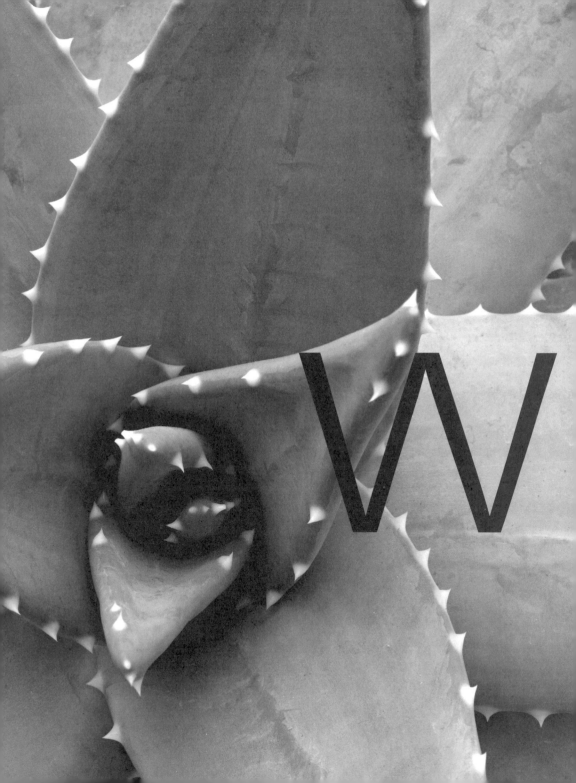

WAKAME
Refer to SEA VEGETABLES.

WATER
Rain was once considered a good source of clean water but when it is mixed with chemicals and other wastes, it loses its life energy. The scientific data available to us regarding the thick band of pollution that surrounds the earth suggests that rain picks up chemicals, germs and lead etc. as it falls through the atmosphere. Filter it.

Well water contains more minerals. Country wells and mountain streams were also once considered a good source of clean water, but with herbicides, pesticides and nitrates now used widely, they too are compromised. Toxicology research has shown that the 'free radicals' created from nitrites (a major farm toxin) neutralise the body's enzymes, creating an internal environment ripe for degenerative disease. Spring water is filtered through clay or mineral beds, and this may be a good source if the area from which it is collected is uncontaminated.

There are many substances added to our town water to 'enhance' it, including chlorine and fluoride. Chlorine combines with other substances in the water to form chloroform, a highly poisonous cancer-causing chemical. Chlorine evaporates once it comes out of the tap, but chloroform doesn't. Chlorine destroys vitamin E in the body, one of the essential vitamins for proper cardiovascular functioning and reproductive health, as well as good bacteria in the intestinal flora. Prolonged exposure to chlorinated water on the skin may contribute to skin cancer.

We assume that where there is tooth decay there is a shortage of fluoride (which gives a hard surface to teeth and bones) in the water. However, the fluorine (the poisonous substance from which fluoride is derived) in food is very different to the fluoride added to our water. Fluorine in food evaporates with cooking or heating; fluoride in water does not. No convincing scientific evidence has shown that adding fluoride to water results in stronger teeth and bones. It is easy to see how many of us would have toxic levels of fluoride in our bodies, as any packaged product that is made with water (not to mention toothpaste and supplementation of fluoride and tap water) will contain fluoride.

The fluoride added to our water is never found in nature—naturally occurring fluoride is non-toxic. The most concentrated naturally occurring source of fluorine is goats milk. Other good sources are avocado, cabbage, lemongrass, parsley, rice, rye and locally sourced sea vegetables. The fluoride in our water interferes with the proper functioning of the thyroid gland, thereby contributing to weight and height abnormalities. It also inhibits all enzyme systems and compromises the immune system. Queensland is the only state in Australia that doesn't fluoridate its water.

After research, some European countries—such as Belgium and Germany, Sweden, Denmark and Holland—have discontinued fluoridation, and France and Norway never found enough reason to start in the first place. Studies are trying to show that dental health is declining in young people due to increased use of bottled water. I would like to suggest that the increased consumption of highly processed, refined junk food is more likely to be the cause. Acid-forming food (refined sugar, flour, meat and dairy), not lack of fluoridated water, ends up damaging teeth. The National Nutrition Survey from 2001 states: 'The high concentration of carbohydrates in some of these junk-food diets, coupled with snacking . . . and soft drinks means there is more exposure to acid attack for teeth.'

Studies are difficult to interpret, as a deciding factor is the mineral content in the water. If there is adequate calcium in the water, the fluoride will form calcium fluoride, which may be beneficial.

Much of our waste is not disposed of properly and it too ends up in our waterways, air, food and soil. A variety of other chemicals are added to our water to prevent the pipes from rusting and also to stabilise the water.

There are a number of filters available to help rid our water of these additives and toxins. Purifiers remove suspended material but leave minerals and other water-soluble substances that may be toxic. Charcoal filters remove toxins and wastes that aren't water-soluble, but leave the dangerous water-soluble toxins, such as fluoride and nitrates. If the water is devoid of these nasties, this system works well. Distillers evaporate water as nature does, but leave hydrocarbons if they are present, and they often are. Reverse-osmosis removes almost all toxins, gases and minerals, leaving you with almost completely pure water. The above systems come in a variety of forms, including jugs, taps or shower nozzle attachments, bottled water and clay pots.

Alkaline water is a great way to alkalise your system.

Much of the chemicals and pollutants found in our waterways prevent your body from doing its job. Your kidneys, liver and adrenals become busy filtering the contaminants, thereby preventing the organs from performing their job properly. The result is that there is now an increase in toxic overload—degenerative diseases, compromised immune function, liver insufficiencies and mental health issues. Parasites are not bothered by chlorination or filtering. Our tap water is also potentially contaminated with other harmful organisms such as viruses and bacteria.

WEIGHT LOSS

Permanent weight loss requires a lifetime commitment to a healthier lifestyle. Getting to know yourself spiritually, physically and emotionally is essential for weight loss. It is important not to feel deprived, which is why it is critical to know what you *can* eat as well as what to avoid. Try to view your weight loss as improving the health of your whole body, not just the way you look.

Obesity has also been linked to food sensitivities and allergies, probably due to insufficient liver function caused by eating too many animal fats and heavy, complex foods.

Helpful foods

- fruits that are low in carbohydrates and kilojoules—apples, rockmelon, grapefruit, strawberries and watermelon
- lemons, limes and grapefruits eaten with the seeds and a little of the inner peel is an excellent weight loss remedy—squeeze a whole lemon in some warm water each morning but avoid if you have ulcers or too much acid in the stomach
- GLA (gamma linolenic acid) is very important for weight loss and great for those who have or are consuming excessive amounts of animal protein—spirulina is the richest source and its nutrients are easy to digest and absorb (it also helps cleanse the body of waste from animal products); wheatgrass and chlorella are great sources too
- wheatgrass reduces appetite
- watercress is fabulous for weight loss
- daikon (Chinese white radish) helps the liver to process fats
- pickles and sauerkraut assist in the absorption of fats, although these should be eaten only in small amounts due to their high salt and vinegar content—a raw food such as pickles or sauerkraut may be eaten any time you're eating a cooked food
- bitter foods, including rye, amaranth, quinoa, oats, lettuce, celery, asparagus, shallots and rocket
- chia seeds will swell in your stomach, keeping you feeling full for longer
- thanks to their medium chain fatty acids, coconut water, milk and oil are great for aiding weight loss
- hummus is a nice snack
- moderate avocado consumption if you already have a high dietary fat background
- protein sources, such as fish and legumes, can increase your metabolism by 30 per cent

- complex carbohydrates such as wholegrains, legumes, fruit and vegetables, nuts and seeds become sweeter the more you chew them and should make up the majority of your diet.

Foods to avoid

- processed foods and animal products
- refined flour, sugar and salt, as they upset metabolism and digestion
- deep-fried foods and those heavy in oil—nuts, seeds and avocados are to be eaten occasionally only
- packaged foods and drinks—and of course all junk food
- eggs are difficult to digest and slow down the function of the liver—eat only two a week and be sure they are free-range or organic
- eating too many fats makes the liver sluggish, increasing the load on the stomach and pancreas, therefore reduce fats from animals (dairy and red meat); goats milk is the only recommended dairy as it normalises weight
- refined and processed oils—gaining weight from fats is twice as likely as gaining weight from eating protein or complex carbohydrates
- avoid artificial sweeteners—they increase appetite and cause digestive problems
- limit sweet and salty foods—salty foods promote fluid in the body and tend to make us crave sweet foods
- go easy on bananas, cherries, corn, dates, dried fruit, figs, grapes, green peas, pears, pineapple, sweet potatoes, potatoes and white rice; eat any carbohydrates for lunch, not at your evening meal
- alcohol.

Herbal medicine

- gymnema for sugar cravings by balancing blood sugar

- St Mary's thistle, dandelion root and schisandra for liver support, thereby aiding digestion
- astragalus improves nutrient absorption, and is also a great energy booster
- cayenne, cinnamon and ginger for digestion and metabolism of fat
- fennel removes fat from the intestinal tract, has slimming properties and is an appetite suppressant
- fenugreek dissolves fat in the liver
- bladderwrack regulates weight loss and low thyroid gland function
- ginger, cloves, cumin, fennel and cayenne increase energy and metabolism
- yarrow, parsley, dandelion leaf, corn silk (inside silky part of corn), celery and alfalfa seeds, as teas help with fluid retention
- green tea, ginger and fenugreek aid digestion and metabolism.

Supplements

- psyllium husks cut down hunger pain as they are a bulking agent—drink with a couple of glasses of water half an hour before meals; they are also a good source of fibre and help with blood sugar levels
- chromium picolinate reduces sugar cravings and is available as a supplement
- kelp aids in weight loss and is available as a supplement, in powder or tablets
- lecithin breaks down fat so it can be removed from the body
- vitamin C speeds up metabolism, thereby helping you burn more kilojoules
- essential fatty acids such as salmon, tuna, flaxseed and evening primrose oil—available as supplements—all help control appetite
- spirulina stabilises blood sugar and is a great source of useable protein—when you're feeling stressed, blend with soy/rice milk, honey or rice syrup and fruit to replace a meal.

Lifestyle factors

- don't be so concerned with kilojoule counting—concentrate on eating a balanced, wholefood diet
- drink eight glasses of pure water daily—don't drink it cold, always at room temperature, as cold water slows down digestion; and try not to drink with meals, as this also messes up digestion
- eat simply and enjoy your food
- fall in love
- follow your heart
- alcohol makes you fat, as it interferes with the burning of fat from fatty deposits
- avoid constipation by eating more fibre
- exercise helps to balance blood sugar levels and helps blood and energy to flow freely throughout the body
- sunlight (in moderate amounts only) stimulates hormones, thereby promoting weight loss
- don't eat or drink alcohol after 8 p.m.
- don't eat when stressed—instead have something easy to digest such as broths or miso soup
- chew!—this is very important for proper digestion
- don't have foods you are avoiding in your cupboard—create a pantry that will help you, not make it harder
- don't go food shopping when you are hungry
- avoid crash/fad diets
- you don't have to be skinny—curves are healthy and gorgeous
- evening meals should be the lightest of the day
- in the morning make a tea with any of the following—burdock, dandelion, chamomile or chicory; wheatgrass, spirulina and juices are great in the morning too

- for sugar cravings, drink some licorice tea
- sugar substitutes (which still need to be consumed in moderation) are molasses, rice syrup, barley malt, amasake (pounded rice product), stevia (a herb that is 300 times sweeter than sugar—available from health food stores in a powder or liquid)
- try not to see yourself through others' eyes
- fluid retention results when your body cannot use a food—it is then stored in the tissues and is harder to burn when there is an inadequate amount of certain nutrients, as they are accumulated in the body
- bake, stir-fry, steam or cook in a cast-iron pan—avoid frying.

SEVEN-DAY WEIGHT LOSS PROGRAM

Day 1

Breakfast	1 piece of mountain bread with 1 egg and 1 teaspoon goats cheese or avocado Herbal, black tea or coffee with soy or rice milk A few slices of rockmelon or a pear
Snack	Two corn thins with hummus and alfalfa
Lunch	Salad of watercress or rocket with canned salmon or another sustainably caught fish, sprouts, Spanish onion, toasted sesame seeds, shallots and a small amount of avocado—dress with lemon juice and black pepper or umeboshi vinegar
Snack	Watermelon, yoghurt and chia seeds, and some peppermint tea with honey
Dinner	Pan-fried blue-eyed cod with stir fried veggies (low carb)
Snack	Fruit salad and yoghurt

Day 2

Breakfast	Large freshly squeezed beetroot, carrot and ginger juice Bircher muesli or oats with soy milk or rice milk, chia and sunflower seeds, walnuts and seasonal fruit. Drizzle with flaxseed oil Herbal teas or coffee; water
Snack	Natural muesli bar and fresh mint tea
Lunch	One piece of mountain bread with salmon, English spinach, scraping of miso paste, small amount of soy mayonnaise, grated carrot and beetroot, pepper
Snack	Small handful of unsalted cashews or macadamia nuts
Dinner	Thai fish cakes with a sweet potato mash
Snack	Green tea and some fruit

Day 3

Breakfast	Smoothie with coconut water, spirulina, chia seeds, flaxseed oil, berries and psyllium husks Dandelion coffee with coconut milk
Snack	Fresh grapefruit juice with a little honey
Lunch	Steamed vegetables—broccoli, zucchini, carrots, mushrooms with brown rice and sardines; a little yoghurt is okay
Snack	One piece of mountain bread or 2 corn thins with tahini and raw honey or rice syrup
Dinner	Grilled organic chicken, tofu or fish (sustainably caught) with baked beetroot, red onion, capsicum and mushrooms. Drizzle with a dressing made from tahini, lemon juice or umeboshi vinegar, garlic, sea salt and water
Snack	Goats milk yoghurt and kiwi fruit

Day 4

Breakfast	Baked beans (homemade) on rye sourdough with rocket
	One 30-millilitre wheatgrass juice
	Fresh ginger and mint tea; water
Snack	Kale, celery and carrot juice
Lunch	Homemade fried brown rice with organic tofu and vegetables
Snack	Fruit-flavoured goats yoghurt with 4 walnuts and flaxseed oil, and some green tea
Dinner	Miso soup or organic chicken soup with loads of vegetables
Snack	A handful of strawberries

Day 5

Breakfast	Fruit-free muesli with fruit salad and goats yoghurt
	Dandelion tea with GM-free soy milk
	Carrot juice
Snack	Green tea and a shot of wheatgrass
Lunch	Two pieces of rye or spelt sourdough or a piece of mountain bread with either organic chicken (marinated) or sustainably caught fish and salad
Snack	Corn thins with pumpkin humus and snow pea sprouts
Dinner	Lentil soup with vegetables
Snack	Raw, dark chocolate

Day 6

Breakfast	Stir-fried tofu, mushrooms and kale in coconut oil with ginger and garlic. Stir through some cooked quinoa, coriander leaves and tamari.
Snack	Dandelion coffee with GM-free soy milk and two corn thins with babaganoush and baby spinach

Lunch	Green salad or steamed vegetables with sustainably caught smoked salmon, capers, red onion, toasted sesame seeds, tomato and alfalfa
Snack	One piece of mountain bread with a scrape of avocado and one piece of marinated tofu
Dinner	Baked kingfish and a rocket salad with a lemon dressing, with steamed, baked or stir-fried vegetables
Snack	One health bar or one bliss ball (see recipe, page 165)

Day 7

Breakfast	Scrambled free-range egg with ¼ cup goats feta and one slice of rye sourdough and loads of fresh herbs Fresh beetroot, carrot, celery and ginger juice
Snack	Herbal tea and a pear
Lunch	Quinoa, cannellini and asparagus salad with nuts and seeds Steamed green beans on the side
Snack	Two dates and peppermint tea with a little honey
Dinner	Seafood and vegetable curry and quinoa

See also BLOOD SUGAR, CARDIOVASCULAR HEALTH, DIGESTION, GLUTEN INTOLERANCE, HERBAL TEAS, NUTRIENTS IN FOODS, OILS and SEA VEGETABLES.

WHEAT

This grain calms the mind and helps you focus. It may be used in cases of insomnia, palpitations, symptoms of menopause, irritability and disorders of the nervous system. It is used to treat cases of bed-wetting and diarrhoea. If you are overweight, eat it in moderation, if at all. If you have allergies, it should be eaten with caution. Refined wheat is to be avoided, and spelt is easier to digest and probably better for us than our modern wheat grain.

See also SPELT and WHOLEGRAINS.

WHEATGRASS

The vitality derived from wheatgrass juice is remarkable. Just 30 millilitres (one shot) of freshly squeezed juice contains as much nutritional value as approximately 1 kilogram of fresh green vegetables. You need to 'press' wheatgrass, not put it through a fast juicer, as the heat from the revolutions will destroy its enzymes. There are machines available for pressing grasses and sprouts. This juice is a complete food, an abundant source of B vitamins that includes vitamins C, E and carotene. These vitamins work to successfully destroy free radicals, which can lead to the degeneration of the immune system, and the body as a whole.

Wheatgrass juice has a long tradition as a cleanser of blood, organs and the gastrointestinal tract. Wheatgrass is different to wheat, as one is a green vegetable and the other a grain. The grass contains no gluten and is therefore no more allergenic than spinach or lettuce. Wheatgrass juice will detoxify the body by increasing the elimination of hardened mucus and solidified faecal matter. Its high enzyme content helps dissolve tumours.

The bio-available chlorophyll found in wheatgrass juice can protect us from carcinogens like no other food or medicine. Given that the liver is the main organ of detoxification in the body, it is important to note that chlorophyll stimulates and regenerates it. Both chlorophyll and haemoglobin (red blood cells) are molecularly similar. The only actual difference is that the central element in chlorophyll is magnesium and in haemoglobin it is iron. So chlorophyll has been shown to build red blood cells after ingestion.

Wheatgrass is available as a fresh plant, juice, or dried in a tablet or powder. Fresh wheatgrass contains five enzymes. Dried does not contain all these enzymes but has the advantage of fibre. One 30 millilitre shot is a good daily habit.

WHOLEGRAINS

Wholegrains are necessary for proper digestion, to calm the nervous system, to encourage sleep, to satisfy hunger and taste (thereby decreasing cravings), to build energy and endurance, and to help elimination, good reflexes, a long memory and clear thinking. Wholegrains require a different digestive procedure from refined grains. Many grains are mildly acidic and most diseases involve an overly acidic condition in the blood. Saliva is alkaline, so chew grains well, as saliva is needed to digest them properly. Soak your grains overnight to increase their digestibility.

Those who have trouble chewing should eat their wholegrains as cereals, puffs, flours or meals.

See also AMARANTH, BARLEY, BUCKWHEAT, CORN, KAMUT, MILLET, OATS, QUINOA, RICE, RYE, SPELT and WHEAT.

WINTER

This is the season to warm your internal body as the surface of your body cools. It is a time to rest, practise techniques such as meditation and yoga, and store energy. Your kidneys are most sensitive now and, as your ears are related to the health of your kidneys, listening and hearing are heightened. The foundation for your body, kidneys control the lower part of your body and your sexual organs. They also promote energy and warmth.

According to traditional Chinese medicine, salty and bitter foods are energetically 'sinking' flavours that help with storage and bring body heat deeper and lower, making you notice the cold less. Excess salt, however, will tighten the kidneys and bladder, causing coldness and fluid retention, and weakening all organs.

Your kidneys store fear, so if they're not healthy, it is common to feel insecure, anxious, alone and isolated throughout this season. A person with healthy kidneys can accomplish a lot without stress. Fear, anxiety and insecurity in excess block loving experiences (due to the kidneys' relationship with the heart) and make you undependable, agitated, ungrounded and nervous.

A person with poor kidney health will most likely be weak, have thin hair and eyebrows or hair loss, chronic split ends and premature greying, weak knees, loose teeth, lower back pain, hearing loss, ear infections and disease, reproductive or sexual issues and poor bone density, be sexually promiscuous, frequently urinate and/or have incontinence, dribbling urine and other urinary and seminal control issues. There will also be decreased growth of both the body and mind.

Helpful foods

- hearty soups, wholegrains, roasted nuts, dried foods, small dark beans such as adzuki, locally sourced sea vegetables, oysters and parsley—these strengthen the kidneys in winter
- millet, barley, organic tofu, black beans and other beans, kudzu, wheatgerm, potato, black sesame seeds, almond milk, sardines, crab and clams are also helpful for strengthening
- bitter foods such as lettuce, watercress, endive, turnip, celery, asparagus, alfalfa, rye, oats, quinoa and amaranth—bitter foods are said to put joy in our hearts
- salty foods such as miso, soy sauce, sea vegetables, sea salt, millet and barley, and anything where salt is added
- ginger to improve circulation
- you can use a little more good quality oil in winter
- dark foods to nourish.

Foods to avoid

- too many warming foods such as lamb, cinnamon, cloves, ginger and chillies
- excess salt.

Herbal medicine

- rosehips and raspberry leaf as a tea
- rehmannia, schisandra, gravel root, marshmallow root, asparagus root, nettle and aloe vera gel
- bitter herbs such as burdock, horsetail, chaparral and chicory root—this last one is available roasted and ground for use as a coffee substitute.

Supplements

- spirulina and chlorella nurture the kidneys, as do bee pollen and royal jelly (check for allergy).

Lifestyle factors

- use longer cooking methods with more water over a lower temperature
- avoid warming substances, such as coffee, alcohol and cigarettes
- avoid overeating
- avoid exposure to environmental toxins
- avoid marijuana, sweet foods, too much protein, rich diets and too much work.

See also AUTUMN, ORGANS AND ASSOCIATED EMOTIONS, SPRING and SUMMER.

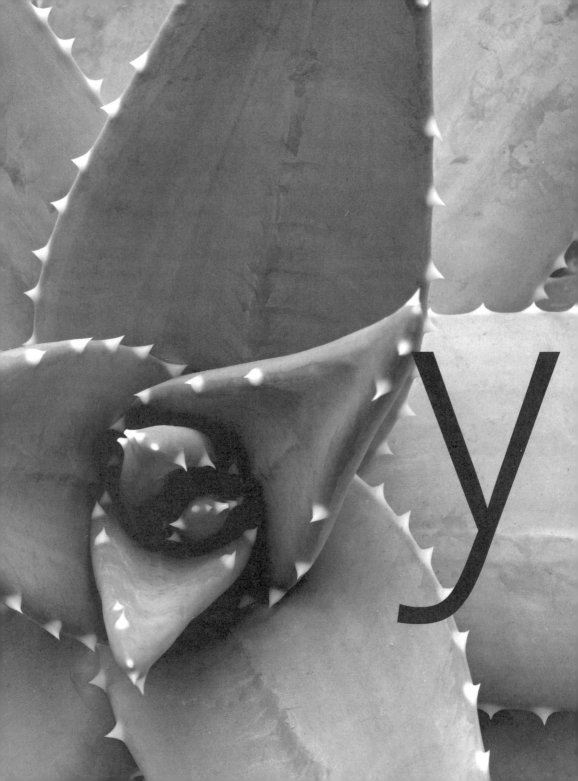

YEAST

Yeast is highly nutritious, containing all the B vitamins (check the list of ingredients on the yeast container to ensure B12 is present) and sixteen of the 22 amino acids. It is high in phosphorus and contains at least fourteen minerals. The high content of phosphorus may deplete the body of calcium, which is why some manufacturers now add calcium to their yeast. It is mostly made up of protein. Be sure to buy a food-grade nutritional yeast known as 'primary' yeast. Bakers' yeast contains live cells that cause depletion of essential vitamins and other essential nutrients. These live cells are not present in nutritional yeast, which is very high in niacin. If candida is present, avoid yeast, as it may induce unhealthy amounts of candida-type yeasts in the body. Yeasted bread may contribute to bloating, indigestion and candida, so buy sourdough. Yeast is also in many other foods such as crackers, packaged foods, cakes and pizza.

See also BREAD and CANDIDA.

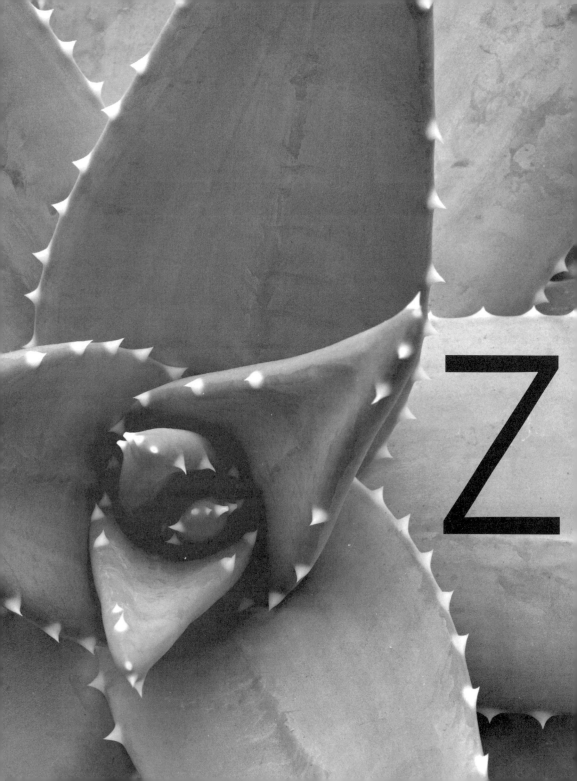

Z

ZINC

This is vitally important for prostate gland function, reproductive organ health, acne control and the regulation of activity of oil glands, protein synthesis and collagen formation, healthy immune system promotion, wound healing, acuity of taste and smell, liver protection from chemical damage, bone formation and to maintain proper concentration of vitamin E. Its levels within your body are depleted by diarrhoea, kidney disease, diabetes, consumption of fibre (causes zinc to be excreted through the intestinal tract), perspiration, hard water, phytates (found in grains and legumes), and iron supplantation, which interferes with zinc absorption.

Sure signs of a deficiency are loss of taste and smell; fingernails that become brittle, thin, peel or develop white spots; acne; fatigue; growth impairment; hair loss; high cholesterol; impaired night vision; impotence; low immunity; poor memory; infertility; prostate trouble; diabetes; skin lesions; and slow wound healing.

Helpful foods
- wheatgerm, miso, pumpkin seeds, oysters, alfalfa, sardines, legumes, mushrooms, pecans, organic soybeans, sunflower seeds and wholegrains.

Supplements
- it is more effective to take liquid zinc, as it is absorbed by the body faster and easier than a tablet. Take it in the evening.

The energetics
of food

Food	Flavour	Functions	Indications
Apples	Sweet	Clear heat and relieve irritability; produce body fluid and relieve thirst; tonify the spleen to stop diarrhoea	Irritability; thirst; indigestion; loose stools or diarrhoea; over-consumption of alcohol
Apricots	Sweet	Produce body fluids and moisten the lungs; regulate lung qi and regulate cough	Dry mouth or thirst; dry cough; asthma
Bananas	Sweet	Clear heat and produce body fluid; nourish yin and moisten dryness	Irritability; thirst or dry mouth; constipation; haemorrhoids
Bitter melons	Bitter	Clear heat and summer irritability; clean liver heat and brighten eyes	Fever; sore throat; thirst; irritability; diabetes; red, painful eyes
Black sesame	Sweet	Nourishes the liver and kidney; moisturises the interior	Dizziness, weakness or dry stools due to liver and kidney yin deficiency; early greying of hair
Cabbages	Sweet	Tonify the spleen and stomach	Weak spleen and stomach; indigestion; peptic ulcers

Food	Flavour	Functions	Indications
Carrots	Sweet	Tonify the spleen and stomach and promote digestion; tonify the liver yin (blood) and brighten the eyes	Food stagnation; dry eyes, night blindness, cataract etc. due to liver blood deficiency; slow eruption of measles
Celery	Sweet and pungent	Clears liver heat and suppresses liver yang; promotes diuresis and excretes damp	Hypertension; vertigo, headache, flushed face or red eyes due to liver heat; painful, hot urination, blood in urine
Chestnuts	Sweet	Strengthen spleen and stomach; tonify kidney; benefit the muscles and bones	Regurgitation or diarrhoea due to stomach or spleen deficiency; soreness of waist and weakness of legs due to kidney deficiency
Chillies	Pungent	Strengthen the stomach; expel cold and dry dampness; induce perspiration	Cold pain in the abdomen, regurgitation, watery vomiting, diarrhoea; cold; arthritis
Chrysanthemum	Sweet	Clears the liver and brightens the eyes; calms liver yang and suppresses liver wind; expels external wind–heat	Red, painful or tearing eyes; hypertension
Coconuts	Sweet	Clear heat; produce body fluid to relieve thirst	Irritability; thirst; dry cough
Cucumbers	Sweet	Clear heat and summer heat; cool blood; eliminate phlegm	Fever; thirst; irritability; cough with phlegm; blood in urine and stools

Food	Flavour	Functions	Indications
Eggplants	Sweet	Clear heat, cool blood	Blood in stools; haemorrhoids; blood stasis
Garlic	Pungent	Expels cold; strengthens the stomach and promotes digestion; relieves toxicity; kills parasites	Nausea, vomiting due to cold in stomach; poor appetite, indigestion; diarrhoea or dysentery; shellfish poisoning; intestinal worms
Ginger	Pungent	Relieves vomiting, warms the lungs and relieves coughing; detoxes seafood and some herbs; induces perspiration to reduce external wind–cold	Nausea, vomiting due to cold in stomach; morning sickness; coughing due to wind–cold; seafood poisoning and allergic reaction
Ginseng	Sweet and bitter	Strongly tonifies heart, stomach, spleen and lungs; produces body fluids to relieve thirst; benefits heart qi to calm shen	Qi deficiency syndrome (lung, heart, spleen or stomach)
Glutinous rice	Sweet	Tonifies the spleen, lungs and stomach qi	Loose stools or diarrhoea due to weak spleen and stomach
Grapes	Sweet	Tonify qi and blood, liver and kidneys; benefit tendons and bones; promote diuresis	Tiredness, palpitations, night sweats due to blood and qi deficiency; weak and/or sore lower back or knees due to kidney deficiency; scanty urine; oedema

Food	Flavour	Functions	Indications
Honey	Sweet	Tonifies the spleen and stomach; nourishes the lungs to relieve cough; moisturises the intestines to relax bowel	Spleen and stomach qi deficiency; blood deficiency
Kiwifruits	Sweet	Clear heat and produce body fluid; tonify stomach yin to promote digestion	Irritability; thirst; poor appetite, nausea or vomiting
Lemons	Sour	Clear heat; produce body fluid to relieve thirst; regulate stomach to produce digestion	Irritability; thirst; indigestion; poor appetite; nausea or vomiting
Licorice root	Sweet	Detoxification; harmonises herbs	Food or herb poisoning; adjusts taste and effect of herbs
Lotus seeds	Sweet and sour	Tonify spleen to relieve diarrhoea; tonify kidney to preserve jing; tonify heart to calm shen	Diarrhoea, poor appetite due to spleen deficiency; seminal emission; leucorrhoea due to kidney deficiency; palpitation; insomnia
Lychees	Sweet	Tonify qi and blood	Poor appetite; loose stools due to weak spleen; dizziness; palpitation due to blood deficiency
Mung beans	Sweet	Clear heat and toxins; promote urination	Toxic or summer heat syndrome; oedema; herb poisoning

Food	Flavour	Functions	Indications
Mushrooms	Sweet	Tonify the spleen and stomach; moisten dryness	Weak spleen and stomach; dry cough; insufficient lactation
Oranges	Sweet and sour	Regulate stomach qi and promote digestion; moisten lungs to relieve cough	Fullness in chest and stomach; poor appetite, nausea or vomiting; cough with dry phlegm; dry mouth and thirst; over-consumption of alcohol
Peanuts	Sweet	Moisten the lungs; strengthen the spleen to stop bleeding	Dry cough; hypogalactia, and bleeding diseases including haemophilia
Pepper	Pungent	Expels cold; eliminates phlegm; relieves toxicity	Cold pain in the abdomen, regurgitation, watery vomiting, diarrhoea; food poisoning and stagnation; phlegm
Pineapples	Sweet	Tonify the stomach yin and produce body fluid; promote diuresis	Irritability; thirst; poor appetite, nausea or vomiting; scanty urination, oedema
Potatoes	Sweet	Tonify the spleen and stomach	Weak spleen and stomach; indigestion; peptic ulcers
Shallots	Pungent	Warm yang and expel internal cold; relieve toxicity; induce perspiration	Mild, external wind–cold syndrome; nasal congestion; abdominal pain due to internal cold; seafood poisoning

Food	Flavour	Functions	Indications
Spinach	Sweet	Clears heat and produces body fluid; moistens dryness and relaxes the bowels; nourishes the liver and brightens the eyes	Polydipsia due to diabetes; dry stools or constipation; dizziness; dim eyesight due to blood deficiency; scurvy; anaemia
Tofu	Sweet	Nourishes yin; benefits the stomach	Diabetes and alcohol poisoning
Tomatoes	Sweet	Clear heat and produce body fluid; cool blood and nourish yin	Thirst, dry throat; dry eyes, night blindness; gum or nose bleeding
Walnuts	Sweet	Tonify kidney and relieve spontaneous seminal emissions; warm the lungs to relieve asthma; moisturise the intestines to relax the bowels	Asthma; frequent urination; impotence and seminal emissions; dry stools
Watermelons	Sweet	Clear heat to relieve irritability; produce body fluids to relieve thirst; promote diuresis	Irritability or thirst due to summer heat; mouth ulcers; scanty or dark urine
Wheat	Sweet	Nourishes the heart and kidney; clears heat and relieves thirst	Hysteria, dysphoria, diabetes etc.
White radishes	Sweet and pungent	Promote digestion; clear phlegm heat; detoxification	Fullness in stomach; poor appetite; belching with foul smell; cough with yellow sputum; diabetes; food poisoning

List of herbs

albizia (*Albizia lebbeck*)—anti-allergic, reduces cholesterol, antimicrobial

aloe vera (*Aloe barbadensis*)—immune-enhancing, antiviral, anti-inflammatory, antitumour, topically for healing wounds, burns, herpes and cuts

andrographis (*Andrographis paniculata*)—immune-enhancing, anti-inflammatory, protects liver, antioxidant, antiplatelet, expels or destroys worms, stops itching, bitter tonic, boosts bile production. *Caution: avoid in pregnancy*

asparagus (*Asparagus racemosus*)—tonic, reduces spasms and diarrhoea, diuretic, increases breast milk, sexual tonic

astragalus (*Astragalus membranaceus*)—reduces physical effects of stress, general tonic, heart tonic, lowers blood pressure, antioxidant, increases secretion and elimination of urine

bacopa (*Bacopa monnieri*)—tonic for nervous system, mild sedative, anti-anxiety, enhances brain function

baical skullcap (*Scutellaria baicalensis*)—anti-inflammatory, anti-allergic, antimicrobial

bilberry (*Vaccinium myrtillus*)—antioxidant, anti-inflammatory, antioedema, protects vascular system, for proper functioning of visual processes

black cohosh (*Cimicifuga racemosa*)—modulates oestrogen, uterine tonic, reduces spasms, reduces rheumatism. *Caution: avoid during pregnancy and lactation*

black haw (*Virburnum prunifolium*)—uterine sedative, anti-asthmatic, reduces elevated blood pressure, secretions, discharges and bronchial spasms

black walnut (*Juglans nigra*)—reduces spasms, oestrogen-modulating, uterine tonic, antirheumatic

bladderwrack (*Fucus vesiculosus*)—weight-reducing, stimulates thyroid, soothes and protects inflamed internal tissue

blue cohosh (*Caulophyllum thalictroides*)—uterine and ovarian tonic, stimulates uterine contractions, stimulates and normalises menstrual flow, reduces spasms. *Caution: avoid in pregnancy and lactation*

boswellia (*Boswellia serrata*)—temporary relief of pain and inflammation of arthritis, osteoarthritis and rheumatism

buchu (*Agathosma betulina*)—urinary tract antiseptic, mild diuretic

bugleweed (*Lycopus virginicus*)—reduces heart rate, mild sedative, normalises overactive thyroid. *Caution: avoid in pregnancy, lactation and hypothyroidism and associated problems*

bupleurum (*Bupleurum falcatum*)—anti-inflammatory, protects heart, reduces cough, aids skin in elimination of toxins and promotes perspiration, regulates menstruation, improves poor liver function

burdock (*Arctium lappa*)—mild diuretic and laxative, reduces all types of skin eruptions

calendula (*Calendula officinalis*)—eye problems, externally for wound healing, anti-inflammatory, antimicrobial, topically antiviral and antifungal, enhances lymphatic system. *Caution: may cause an allergic reaction in susceptible types*

California poppy (*Eschscholtzia californica*)—anti-anxiety, mild sedative, reduces pain

cat's claw (*Uncaria tomentosa*)—immune-enhancing, anti-inflammatory, antioxidant. *Caution: use with caution in pregnancy and lactation*

celery seed (*Apium graveolens*)—increases secretion and elimination of urine, anti-inflammatory, reduces symptoms of arthritis and gout, urinary tract antiseptic, rheumatic pain. *Caution: use with caution in kidney disorders*

chamomile, German (*Matricaria recutita*)—anti-inflammatory, reduces spasms, mild sedative, anti-ulcer, externally for healing wounds and cuts, aids skin in the elimination of toxins and promotes perspiration, digestive disorders especially associated with nervous system, inflamed and sore eyes. *Caution: may cause an allergic reaction*

chaparral (*Larrea tridentata*)—cleans blood, antiseptic, reduces excess mucus, antitumour, diuretic, antibiotic, destroys or eliminates parasites

chaste tree (*Vitex agnus-castus*)—relief of premenstrual tension, menstrual pain and symptoms caused by irregularities of the menstrual cycle; increases breast milk, balances female hormones. *Caution: avoid when taking contraceptive pill*

chen pi mandarin peel (*Citrus reticulata*)—reduces cough, eliminates excess mucus, improves digestion, stimulant, aids stomach

chickweed succus (*Stellaria media*)—soothes and protects inflamed internal tissue, reduces secretions, discharge and peptic ulcers; topically for cuts, wounds, itching, irritation, eczema and psoriasis; internally for rheumatism

cinnamon quills (*Cinnamomum zeylandica*)—soothes and protects inflamed internal tissue, relaxes stomach to support digestion. *Caution: may cause allergy*

citrus seed extract (*Citrus* spp.)—stimulant, aids digestion, reduces cough, parasites and excess mucus

corn silk (*Zea mays*)—increases secretion and elimination of urine, soothes and protects inflamed urinary tract tissue, improves kidney function

corydalis (*Corydalis ambigua*)—for heart and nerve problems, neuralgia pain, period pain, headache, sedative

couch grass (*Agropyron repens*)—soothes irritations of the urinary tract, soothes and protects inflamed urinary tract tissue

cramp bark (*Viburnum opulus*)—reduces cramping, mild sedative, reduces secretions and discharge, reduces blood pressure

crataeva (*Crataeva nurvala*)—breaks down stones and other hard masses, bladder tonic, anti-inflammatory

damiana (*Turnera diffusa*)—mild laxative, soothes nervous system, increases testosterone

dandelion (*Taraxacum officinale*)—boosts bile production, increases secretion and elimination of urine (especially the leaf), mild laxative, reduces rheumatism, tonic. *Caution: avoid in bile duct closure; may cause allergy*

dan shen (*Salvia miltiorrhiza*)—for high blood pressure, palpitations, acute or chronic liver disease, poor circulation associated with diabetes, skin disorders; promotes healing of fractures and other injuries

devil's claw (*Harpagophytum procumbens*)—anti-inflammatory, reduces pain, bitter tonic, reduces rheumatism

dong quai (*Angelica sinensis*)—anti-inflammatory, mild laxative, relief of menstrual cramps and pain and premenstrual tension, helps with anaemia, reduces platelets. *Caution: avoid in pregnancy, haemorrhage and heavy periods*

echinacea (*Echinacea purpurea* and *E. angustifolia*)—immune modulator and enhancer; blood cleanser; anti-inflammatory; topically for wound healing; stimulates saliva; improves lymphatic system; relief of symptoms of colds, influenza and other mild upper respiratory infections. *Caution: risk of allergic reaction to echinacea is very small, especially to the roots since these are free of pollens; contraindicated with immunosuppressant medication (e.g. for transplant patients) so short-term therapy only is suggested*

elder (*Sambucus nigra*)—reduces catarrh, aids skin in the elimination of toxins and promotes perspiration

elecampane (*Inula helenium*)—children's bronchial cough, fever, respiratory complaints, aids skin in the elimination of toxins and promotes perspiration, antibacterial, reduces spasms especially in bronchioles

eyebright (*Euphrasia officinalis*)—reduces secretions, catarrh and discharge; anti-inflammatory; tonic for mucous membranes

false unicorn root (*Chamaelirium luteum*)—uterine and ovarian tonic, modulates oestrogen

fennel (*Foeniculum vulgare*)—reduces spasms, modulates oestrogen, antimicrobial, helps remove excess phlegm from chest, calming, relieves flatulence, increases the flow of breast milk, aids weight loss. *Caution: may cause a reaction in those allergic to celery, carrots and mugwort*

fenugreek (*Trigonella foenum-graecum*)—appetite stimulant, increases breast milk, anti-inflammatory, reduces high blood sugar and cholesterol, soothes and protects inflamed internal tissue. *Caution: avoid in hypothyroidism; may interact with the drug Warfarin*

feverfew (*Tanacetum parthenium*)—anti-inflammatory, anti-allergic, bitter tonic, stimulates and normalises menstrual flow, increases breast milk, expels or destroys worms, temporary relief of migraines and tension headaches

garlic (*Allium sativum*)—relieves mucus congestion, improves peripheral circulation, helps maintain integrity of capillaries, supportive of dietary measures to help maintain healthy blood lipid levels or cholesterol levels. *Caution: use with caution in patients taking anti-platelet drugs; contraindicated with Warfarin if dose greater than 5 g fresh garlic per day, unless under close supervision; discontinue intake 10 days before surgery; not advised for patients taking HIV protease inhibitors such as Saquinavir*

gentian (*Gentiana lutea*)—bitter tonic, stimulates gastric juices, aids skin in the elimination of toxins and promotes perspiration, stimulates saliva. *Caution: avoid in gastric disorders such as gastric and peptic ulcers, acid reflux and inflammation of the gut*

ginger (*Zingiber officinale*)—reduces nausea and vomiting, calms the stomach, peripheral circulatory stimulant, aids digestion, reduces spasms, aids with morning sickness, promotes sweating, anti-inflammatory, relieves travel sickness, reduces pain in body due to coldness, aids skin in the elimination of toxins and promotes perspiration. *Caution: may interfere with pharmaceutical drugs; avoid in cases of gastric disorders such as reflux and ulcers*

ginkgo (*Ginkgo biloba*)—antioxidant, protects neurotransmittors, circulatory stimulant, enhances brain function. *Caution: contraindicated with Warfarin unless under close supervision; avoid taking with aspirin or haloperidol (reduce dose of haloperidol if necessary in conjunction with prescribing physician)*

globe artichoke (*Cynara cardunculus* var. *scolymus*)—protects and restores proper liver function, bitter tonic, reduces high cholesterol, stops vomiting, aids skin in the elimination of toxins and promotes perspiration, blood cleanser, increases secretion and elimination of urine. *Caution: avoid in gall bladder disorders*

golden seal (*Hydrastis canadensis*)—reduces haemorrhage, restorative action on mucous membranes, bitter tonic, anti-inflammatory, blood cleanser, topically for wounds, antibacterial, may induce uterine contractions. *Caution: may reinforce effects of drugs that displace the protein binding of bilirubin*

grape complex (*Vitis vinifera*)—powerful antioxidant

gravel root (*Eupatorium purpureum*)—softens and removes kidney stones and gravel

gymnema (*Gymnema sylvestre*)—helps maintain normal and healthy blood sugar levels, reduces elevated cholesterol, reduces weight, helps with sugar and carbohydrate cravings. *Caution: particular care should be exercised when taking insulin or oral hypoglycaemic drugs*

hawthorn berry and leaf (*Crataegus monogyna*)—supports cardiovascular system and circulatory functions, assists in maintenance of peripheral circulation, reduces blood pressure, corrects heart rhythms, antioxidant, stabilises collagen. *Caution: may potentiate the action of hypotensive medication; due to tannins, consume at least two hours away from ingestion of mineral supplements*

horse chestnut (*Aesculus hippocastanum*)—anti-inflammatory, tonic for veins, reduces bruising. *Caution: avoid applying to broken skin*

horseradish (*Armoracia rusticana*)—nasal and bronchial dilator, relieves symptoms of 'flu and fever, reduces flatulence

horsetail (*Equisetum arvense*)—relieves urinary tract disorders such as kidney stones, bed wetting and cystitis; healing for lung damage; breaks down lumps, especially in prostate; relieves gout; reduces or stops external bleeding; increases secretion and elimination of urine; reduces secretions and discharge, such as those from sex organs and wounds

Korean ginseng (*Panax ginseng*)—reduces physical effects of stress, immune-modulating, heart tonic, brain tonic, male tonic, cancer preventative.

Caution: avoid with heavy periods, acute asthma, nose bleeds or acute infections

ladies mantle (*Alchemilla vulgaris*)—anti-inflammatory, topically for wounds, reduces secretions and discharge, stimulates and normalises menstrual flow

lemon balm (*Melissa officinalis*)—calms stomach, reduces spasms, mild sedative, topically antiviral, aids skin in the elimination of toxins and promotes perspiration

licorice (*Glycyrrhiza glabra*)—anti-inflammatory, reduces peptic ulcers, protects mucous membranes, adrenal tonic, removes excess mucus from respiratory system, reduces cough, mild laxative. *Caution: not to be taken in cirrhosis of liver, severe kidney disorders, high blood pressure, oedema; may interfere with contraceptive pill; best to avoid during pregnancy; may interfere with prednisone and other steroids*

meadowsweet (*Filipendula ulmaria*)—anti-inflammatory, antacid, mild urinary antiseptic, reduces secretions and discharge, helps with digestive disorders. *Caution: avoid if salicylate sensitive*

Mexican valerian (*Valeriana edulis*)—reduces spasms, temporary relief of insomnia, relief of nervous tension and mild anxiety

motherwort (*Leonurus cardiaca*)—menstrual and uterine conditions related to anxiety or depression, sedative for pregnant women, heart palpitations and other heart conditions related to anxiety. *Caution: avoid in pregnancy*

mugwort (*Artemisia vulgaris*)—bitter tonic, stimulant, nervous system tonic, stimulates and normalises menstrual flow

mullein (*Verbascum thapsus*)—relieves dry cough, topically for wounds, protects irritated or inflamed internal tissue, removes excessive amounts of mucus from the respiratory tract, helps with chest irritations, asthma and bronchitis

myrrh (*Commiphora molmol*)—antimicrobial, antibacterial, anti-inflammatory, topically for wounds, reduces secretions and discharge. *Caution: avoid in pregnancy and excessive uterine bleeding; don't use for extended periods*

neem (*Azadirachta indica*)—antimicrobial, antifungal, antiviral, reduces itching, reduces coughing, cleanses blood, anti-inflammatory, reduces anxiety, normalises blood glucose, immune-enhancing, stimulates and normalises menstrual cycle, reduces the physical effects of stress. *Caution: avoid during pregnancy and when receiving treatment for infertility*

nettle (*Urtica dioica*)—anti-allergic, cleanses blood, reduces or stops external bleeding, reduces rheumatism

oat seed (*Avena sativa*)—soothes nervous system, for skin applications

olive leaf (*Olea europaea*)—antioxidant, bitter tonic, reduces blood pressure

paeonia (*Paeonia lactiflora*)—for menstrual dysfunction, polycystic ovarian disease, muscle cramps, assists memory

passion flower (*Passiflora incarnata*)—reduces anxiety and spasms, helps with insomnia, mild sedative

pau d'arco (*Tabebuia impetiginosa*)—immune-enhancing, antitumour, antibacterial, antifungal, cleanses blood, removes or destroys parasites. *Caution: avoid with anticoagulant therapy and pregnancy*

paw paw leaves (*Papaya carica*)—stimulates appetite and aids digestion, antitumour, used to treat diarrhoea

peppermint (*Mentha* x *piperita*)—reduces spasms, calms stomach, reduces vomiting, anti-microbial (internally and externally), mild sedative, applied topically may reduce itchiness, reduces cough, boosts bile production. *Caution: avoid with oesophageal reflux, gallstones and salicylate sensitivity*

phyllanthus (*Phyllanthus amarus*)—for viral diseases of liver, protects liver, normalises blood sugar

poke root (*Phytolacca decandra*)—anti-inflammatory, immune-enhancing, cleanses blood, aids sinusitis, lymphatic tonic for lumps in breasts and mastitis. *Caution: avoid in pregnancy, lactation, with immunosuppressant drugs and lymphocytic leukaemia*

raspberry leaf (*Rubus idaeus*)—reduces secretions, discharges and diarrhoea; uterine tonic. *Caution: better to avoid in first trimester of pregnancy*

red clover flowers (*Trifolium pratense*)—antitumour, cleanses blood, female reproductive tonic

rehmannia (*Rehmannia glutinosa*)—adrenal tonic, reduces haemorrhage, anti-inflammatory, reduces itch

rhubarb root (*Rheum palmatum*)—reduces secretions and discharges, bitter tonic, mild purgative

sage (*Salvia officinalis*)—reduces spasms, antioxidant, antimicrobial, anti-hydrotic (reduces sweat), reduces secretions and discharges. *Caution: avoid in pregnancy and lactation; do not exceed recommended dosage*

St John's wort (*Hypericum perforatum*)—sedative, relieves pain in nerve endings, for depression, relaxant, sleep disturbances, relieves sciatica, antiviral, anti-inflammatory, antimicrobial, tonic for the nervous system. *Caution: not to be taken with Warfarin, Digoxin, Cyclosporine, Indinavir and related HIV drugs*

St Mary's thistle (*Silybum marianum*)—supportive tonic for the liver and liver function, antioxidant

sarsaparilla (*Smilax ornata*)—anti-inflammatory, cleanses blood, reduces rheumatism, chronic skin disorders

saw palmetto (*Serenoa serrulata*)—anti-inflammatory, reduces spasms, protects against prostate problems, male reproductive system tonic, sexual dysfunction, urinary tract problems

schisandra (*Schisandra chinensis*)—protects liver, counters effects of modern living, antioxidant, nervous system tonic, reduces cough, stimulates uterine contractions, mild antidepressant, reduces physical effects of stress. *Caution: avoid in pregnancy*

senna pods (*Cassia senna*)—stimulating laxative, effective six hours after ingestion. Short-term use is preferable

shepherd's purse (*Capsella bursa-pastoris*)—reduces bleeding, urinary antiseptic

Siberian ginseng (*Eleutherococcus senticosus*)—for physical or emotional stress, exhaustion, depression, long-term illnesses. *Caution: best avoided in acute stage of infection*

skullcap (*Scutellaria lateriflora*)—tonic for nervous system, mild sedative, reduces spasms, depression

thuja (*Thuja occidentalis*)—antimicrobial, antifungal, antiviral, cleans blood. *Caution: not to be used in pregnancy or lactation; use with caution in epilepsy; avoid high doses over a prolonged period*

thyme (*Thymus vulgaris*)—antibacterial, antifungal, antioxidant, antimicrobial, reduces spasms, topically to increase circulation in the skin thus relieving internal pains

tienchi ginseng (*Panax notoginseng*)—reduces bleeding, protects heart, anti-inflammatory, corrects rhythm of the heart, reduces high cholesterol. *Caution: not to be taken in pregnancy*

turmeric (*Curcuma longa*)—anti-inflammatory, antioxidant, calms stomach, cleanses blood, antimicrobial, reduces blood lipids and platelets, liver herb. *Caution: not to be taken with bile duct obstructions; take with caution if gallstones are present*

valerian (*Valeriana officinalis*)—mild sedative, reduces anxiety and spasms

vervain (*Verbena officinalis*)—reduces secretions and discharges, tonic for the nervous system, mild depressant, promotes sweat to eliminate toxins. *Caution: avoid with meals or iron supplementation*

wild cherry bark (*Prunus serotina*)—sedative for a dry cough and whooping cough, mild sedative, reduces secretions and discharges

wild yam (*Dioscorea villosa*)—anti-inflammatory, modulates oestrogen, reduces spasms and rheumatism

willow bark (*Salix alba*)—anti-inflammatory, reduces secretions and discharges, bitter digestive tonic, local antiseptic

willow herb (*Epilobium parviflorum*)—reduces prostate problems

witch-hazel (*Hamamelis virginiana*)—used locally for bruises, wounds and haemorrhoids; reduces secretions and discharges

withania (*Withania somnifera*)—for nervous exhaustion, blood tonic

wormwood (*Artemisia absinthium*)—bitter tonic, destroys or removes worms and parasites. *Caution: not to be taken during pregnancy or lactation; may cause a reaction in those sensitive to ragweed, daisies and chrysanthemums*

yarrow (*Achillea millefolium*)—promotes sweat thereby eliminating toxins, anti-inflammatory, bitter tonic, antimicrobial, reduces bleeding, topically for wounds, reduces fever, stimulates digestion, urinary antiseptic. *Caution: known allergen*

yellow dock (*Rumex crispus*)—relieves chronic skin disease, mild laxative, cleanses blood, promotes bile production and secretions from the gallbladder

zizyphus (*Zizyphus spinosa*)—hypertension, irritability, palpitations, menopausal flushing, nervous exhaustion, anxiety, excessive sweating. *Caution: avoid in pregnancy and lactation; avoid taking for prolonged periods.*

Glossary

agar agar A dried sea vegetable, agar agar is a vegan substitute for gelatine that can be used for setting desserts and some savoury dishes. Sometimes called kanten, it is available in flakes, powder or bars. Gluten-free.

agave A complex sweetener from the cactus of the same name, agave tastes like toffee. It won't send blood sugar levels up. Gluten-free.

amaranth One of the oldest cultivated cereal varieties and the principal foodstuff of the Incas and Aztecs, amaranth is extraordinarily healthy as a cereal or foliage plant due to its high protein content of 16 per cent. Its leaves are popular as either a vegetable or a seasoning. Gluten-free.

amasake A starter called koji converts the starch in rice into a simple sugar, resulting in amasake or fermented sweet rice. This sugar is not as refined as honey, molasses etc.

arame This sea vegetable contains ten times more calcium than milk and 500 times more iodine than shellfish. Keep it in the fridge, soaking in water, and add it to salads or stir-fries as you need it, or add it as a dried ingredient to winter casseroles, grains and soups. Gluten-free.

bancha Twigs from the green tea plant, anti-inflammatory bancha is an antioxidant with a very high calcium content.

dashi Use this stock as a base for making miso. Available in dried form from health food stores and some supermarkets, it consists of shiitake mushrooms, kombu and bonito (fish) flakes. There is also a vegetarian option without the bonito available. Gluten-free.

dulse Rich in iodine and calcium, this sea vegetable can be used in soups or as a condiment.

flaxseed oil Also known as linseed oil, flaxseed oil comes from the seeds of the flax plant. It contains both omega 3 and omega 6 fatty acids, which are needed for good health. Flaxseed oil contains the essential fatty acid alpha-linolenic acid (ALA), which the body converts into eicosapentaenoic acid (EPA) and docosahexaenoic acid (DHA), the omega 3 fatty acids found in fish oil. Gluten-free.

kale A member of the Brassica family, kale is native to the British Isles and the Eastern Mediterranean. There are many varieties of both curly- and smooth-leafed kale. Called *cavolo nero* in Italy, it is rich in antioxidants (some say more than any other veggie) and, when cooked, does not lose volume like silver beet or spinach, but it does need to be cooked longer.

kamut This unadulterated older cereal variety that dates back to ancient Egypt produces grains that are often three times the size of wheat. It is high in protein as well as rich in amino acids and vitamins.

karengo fronds This sea vegetable is rich in vitamins and minerals, including calcium, magnesium and zinc. These bite-sized pieces can be used as a snack straight out of the bag or used in cooking as a garnish for various dishes. Related to arrowroot, kudzu is used instead of cornflour to thicken sauces. It's also used to treat diarrhoea. Available in small rocks or as a powder, it is gluten-free.

kombu A sea vegetable that contains 500 times the iodine of shellfish, kombu is high in protein, iron and calcium. It is available fresh, dried, pickled and frozen. Use it in soups, salads, bean dishes and pickles.

kudzu Related to arrowroot, kudzu root is used to thicken sauces and also to treat diarrhoea and fever.

lecithin granules Lecithin is a naturally occurring fatty substance found in a variety of different foods, such as soybeans, egg yolks and wholegrains. It helps the body utilise certain vitamins, including A, B, E and K. Lecithin granules also help to break down fat and cholesterol into smaller pieces.

linseed oil *see* flaxseed oil

LSA A combination of ground linseeds (flaxseeds), sunflower seeds and almonds.

maca powder *Lepidium meyenii* is a root plant from Peru consumed as a food and for medicinal purposes. It is traditionally used to increase stamina, sexual function and energy and to balance hormones. It is available as a capsule, liquid extract or powder. Maca is often touted as an aphrodisiac.

millet The oldest cultivated variety of cereal in the world, millet is an important basic foodstuff in Africa and Central Asia that is very rich in unsaturated fatty acids and vitamins.

miso paste This fermented soy product is used in soups and sauces. Miso is high in protein and great for balancing gut flora and any other stomach complaint. It is also a diabetic's best friend, as it balances blood sugar. Never boil miso, as the heat will destroy its live enzymes. Generally the lighter coloured pastes like shiro are sweeter, and the darker—genmai and hatcho—are saltier and more pungent. Use the lighter pastes in the warmer weather. Gluten-free.

mochi Pounded 'sweet' or 'glutinous' rice, which is easy to digest, is used for anaemia or depletion.

natto miso A fermented soybean product made from whole cooked soybeans inoculated with *Bacillus subtilis*, it's high in protein and rich in fibre, with very little sodium.

nori You can buy this dried sea vegetable in paper-like sheets. Eat it as a snack or wrap it around rice. Of all the sea vegetables, nori, along with wakame, has the highest protein content and is the easiest to digest. Garnish your vegetables or soups with shredded nori. Or use it instead of flatbread for your wraps. Gluten-free.

oatmeal This is ground oats as opposed to whole oats or oat flakes.

Omega spread Melrose Foods has developed an alternative to margarine and butter. The Omegacare range of table spreads is high in omega 3 oils and very low in saturated fat. They are neither hydrogenated nor heat-treated, contain minimal natural trans fats, have no cholesterol, are non-dairy and are GM-free.

panela Unrefined whole cane sugar, typical of Latin America, panela or rapadura is a solid piece of sucrose and fructose obtained by boiling and evaporating sugarcane juice.

pepitas High in zinc and fibre, the pepita is the inside part of the pumpkin seed.

pomegranate molasses Made by boiling down the juice of a tart variety of pomegranate, this molasses forms a thick, dark brown liquid that is used in dressings and pilafs.

psyllium seed husks These are portions of the seeds of the plant *Plantago ovata*, native to India. Indigestible, they are a source of soluble dietary fibre, used to relieve constipation, irritable bowel syndrome and diarrhoea. Some recent research also indicates they may lower cholesterol and control diabetes. Gluten-free.

quark A type of fresh cheese, quark is made by warming soured milk until the desired degree of denaturation of milk proteins is met, then strained. Traditional quark is not made with rennet. It is soft, white and unaged, similar to some types of *fromage frais*. It is distinct from ricotta, as the latter is made from scalded whey. Quark usually has no added salt and is known for its beneficial effect on the digestive system. Gluten-free.

quinoa This herb grows in the Andes at altitudes in excess of 4000 metres, and its small seeds are rich in vitamins and nutrients. It is used in the same way as grains, and was much prized by the Incas. Gluten-free.

rapadura *see* panela

raw cacao powder Cacao (pronounced ka-kow) beans are the seeds of an Amazonian fruiting tree and the source of all chocolate and cocoa products. As the temperature during processing is never allowed to exceed 40°C, the powder is considered a 'raw' food with all heat-sensitive vitamins, minerals and antioxidants remaining intact, thereby maximising digestion and absorption. It has over 360 per cent more antioxidants than regular cocoa. Gluten-free.

raw honey The concentrated nectar is pure, unheated, unpasteurised and unprocessed. An alkaline-forming food, this type of honey contains ingredients similar to those found in fruits, which become alkaline in the digestive system. Gluten-free.

rice syrup A complex sweetener with the consistency of honey, but not as sweet, rice syrup is made by pounding brown rice. Gluten-free.

semolina The centre part of durum wheat is obtained after processing and separating it. When mixed with flour, it becomes couscous. It's used to make puddings and other desserts, pasta and breakfast cereals. Contains gluten.

shiitake mushrooms If dried, these Japanese mushrooms need to be soaked in hot water and softened. Discard the stems, or save them for stock and keep the water.

spelt The original wheat grain from Persia contains gluten but is easily digested. It is high in protein and has immune-boosting properties.

tahini A paste made of ground, lightly toasted sesame seeds, tahini is available either hulled (that is, the shells have been taken off) or unhulled. The hulled seeds are used to make sesame paste. Gluten-free.

tamari This wheat-free condiment is a good quality soy sauce from Japan. It is made using fermented soybeans and sea salt. Gluten-free.

tempeh A fermented soybean product of Indonesian origin, tempeh is a good source of protein and vitamin B12. Fry it, then add it to stir-fries or salads. Easy to digest, it is gluten-free.

tofu Made from ground cooked soybeans, tofu is an unfermented soy product that is high in protein and calcium. It is great for the spleen and stomach as well as for stabilising blood sugar. Low in fat. Available as firm, soft, silken or smoked. Gluten-free.

umeboshi plums These salty and sour or pickled plums (actually apricots) from Japan are highly alkaline and antibiotic. They are great for digestion. Umeboshi vinegar is used in pickles and sauces, the plums are eaten whole and the paste is used for pickling or as a condiment. Gluten-free.

wakame A sea vegetable, or edible seaweed, it contains four times more iron than beef and, along with nori, is one of the sea vegetables highest in calcium. It has a subtly sweet flavour and is most often served in soups and salads. New studies have found that a compound in wakame known as fucoxanthin can help burn fatty tissue. In Oriental medicine it has been used for blood purification, intestinal strength, skin, hair, reproductive organs and menstrual regularity. Gluten-free.